My World in my Words

Bobby Latheron

Published by New Generation Publishing in 2019

Copyright © Bobby Latheron 2019

First Edition

The author asserts the moral right under the Copyright, Designs and Patents Act 1988 to be identified as the author of this work.

All Rights reserved. No part of this publication may be reproduced, stored in a retrieval system or transmitted, in any form or by any means without the prior consent of the author, nor be otherwise circulated in any form of binding or cover other than that which it is published and without a similar condition being imposed on the subsequent purchaser.

ISBN 978-1-78955-687-2

www.newgeneration-publishing.com

New Generation Publishing

I just want to say thank you to all the staff from espa (my place team) for helping me to do my book.

I want to thank you Angela for sitting with me for my recordings and writing them all down for me.

I want to thank everyone who did a questionnaire for me.

Also what to thank you friends and my family for believing in me, and also Jess for helping me deign my book with me and Kerry.

Also would like to thanks carl for all the work he has done with me and Jenna and his wife.

A big thank you to my family who have supported me through the book and music.

I cant wait for people to start reading it.

Now let's begin the journey

Chapter 1

I have written a book about autism because for one reason I have autism and also for another reason I think people still do not understand about autism and I think it's about time people did!

I have asked people to complete a questionnaire about what they think about autism and how people live their lives with autism.

I am writing about what I think autism is and how I feel about it.

What is my understanding about autism?

To be honest with you I still don't know much about autism and this is why I am writing a book so I know more about autism and for others to know what the meaning of someone living with autism is?

What I think about people with autism? And how it affects people's lives?

I think with people with autism is that they like to know what they are doing and how to reach they goals and also I know when people get let down they can get very upset because they don't understand it but with others they bite they tongue so you get people to like you and don't think of you in another way but sometimes it can be hard and hurtful.

What do I think of me and my autism?

I think I am very nice person sometimes it's hard to say what I want to say because I don't want people to unlike me and that I let people get away with so much because am just a nice person. I know I don't believe in what I want to do because off my old schools and stuff, I always want to be a helping hand, but then you get let down but from now I just know to think about myself before putting people first because I think if you are 50 50 then yes then you both can work together, also I am bubbly to people and sometimes it's hard for me to be in a relationship but don't want to say anything private about my life because it's private between myself and I know one day I will have a nice person in my life one day.

Do I think it is easy for people with autism to get a job?

No it's not easy for people to have a job with autism because they think "ohh they need extra help" so they don't even bother to give you a job which I think it is unfair yes I do think with people with more autism people needs the one to one but people like me who has got mild autism they need to think of those people who want to work and not because of the autism because they are some people with intelligent and talent are brilliant but they have public scare and I think it should not be a bother if they are because even normal people get scared.

Person 1: what is your understanding of autism?

My understanding is that they are many symptoms of autism and some people with autism may require addition support to help them cope with their symptoms.

What you think about people with autism? And how it affects people's lives?

I think every person with autism, is different in their own individual way. They may have difficulty understanding other people's feelings and repetitive behavior and also dislike changes to their routine.

What do you think of me and my autism?

I think that you cope very well with your autism and socialize and communicate with others well.

Do you think it is easy for people with autism to get a job?

I don't think it is easy for people with autism to get a job. Although I feel this is getting better as people are more open to learning more about autism and that people with autism can be excellent at many things, especially if it something they enjoy.

This was finished on 12.03.18

Person 2: what is your understanding of autism?

Autism is a lifelong neuro – developmental condition which affects individuals in very different ways. It can affect social communication processing time and independence levels. As autism is a spectrum condition it affects individuals differently and with different severity.

What you think about people with autism? And how it affects people's lives?

Autism affects everyone differently and the impact on their lives can be very different. Some lead fully independent lives and develop coping strategies others need to be fully supported. I very much enjoy spending time with people on the autism spectrum.

What do you think of me and my autism?

I think you are a very unique and individuals. You are very caring and your autism helps you to understand what others are going through. Autism has not stopped you achieving what you want to you just need a little extra support at times.

Do you think it is easy for people with autism to get a job?

This can be very difficult but with the right support there is no reason a person with autism can't find employment using individuals strengths such as logical thinking or good problem solving stills can be a real benefit to employers.

This was finished on 12.03.18

Family

I live at home with my mam, sometimes my mam's partner stays and my brother and I have two older sisters. I am autistic and my brother has god ADHD. We are two different people. I love shopping and he likes sports so we don't really have anything in common and we fight but if one or another is upset we are always there for each other. I love my two sisters very much and can't thank them enough for what they do for us. They are both married and again, I get along with both of them. We always have good fun and laugh's especially when we go on a family holiday. I can't really ask for a better mam because she's been there for me from good times to bad times and she is my rock and best friend. Also my mam's partner is like a dad to all of us and I feel like I can tell him anything. I also have a niece who I love very much but sometimes I might not seem I show her any love as an uncle because sometimes I don't like the noise when they are crying so I go in my room and i think that could be because due to my autism.

Animals

I love animals like dogs and sheep's I don't really like snakes or anything like snakes. My sister has one dog and my other sister has three dogs. I love my sister's dogs I go for big walks with them and cuddle them. I remember when one of my sister's dogs got attacked it really frightened me so I put my hands in the other dog's mouth and got her out just in time but she is very lucky to be alive.

My future

In the future my dream job would be to play a part on a soap opera like corrie or Emmerdale or even hollyoaks and I would love to do a storyline about how people cope with autism and see how they live with it. I would also love to play a role in an exciting storyline, I would love to go onto big brother to talk to people about autism and how I cope with it, I might not be good in my math or English but I am one of a hell a good actor. I go and see performances on stage and just say to myself, I could do this and fall in love with it. But I have to wait and hopefully someone will see my book and give me the change to act. Also, it that didn't work I would love to be a songwriter. At the moment I am writing songs and also, I would love to become a book author, also I love writing scripts in my own time.

My birthday 2018

I loved all my presents from all my family as I always get really good presents. I got to see a medium which I really needed to hear to think about my future. One of my sisters gives me money which I love and the same to my brother, and then my other sister got me Parma violet gin which I really love with lemonade. I really don't know how people drink tonic water with gin it's just not my thing! My sister also got me other surprise she got me some singing lessons because I love to learn to sing but really just wants to be a songwriter. I went out with autism matters for some food and I was talking to Leanne and Lynne about my singing lessons that I was getting tomorrow because I was really thrilled and excited for tomorrow and when I was telling them where about it was , they were like well journey south brothers live in that area and they said he got a massive studio in his house and I was like whatever yeah as if he will be my singing teacher. The next day I was getting ready for my singing lesson and when my brother dropped me off I thought it was a big house and he had his own studio in his house with different guitars and microphones and I asked if he was journey south and he said yes I am. I was jumpy and nervous. On the 1st June 2018, I finished my own song he sang it. It's just amazing how I can write songs about life and it really got me tearful but also joyful. The song is acoustic because I love acoustic songs and I can't wait to bring it out for people to listen to it and hopefully people will like it. I can't rally thank him enough as he is really good teacher and I can't wait to work on more of my songs with him.

Chapter 2

Person 3: what is your understanding of autism?

Autism is a condition affects the way people communicate and interact with others. It has different effects on different individuals.

What you think about people with autism? And how it affects people's lives?

I think the problem with autism is that other people do not understand it and feel uneasy when having to communicate with autism people. It definitely has an effect on people's lives but you learn to live with it.

What do I think of me and my autism?

I think that you are a very personable young man, realistic in outlook and aware of your autism.

Do I think it is easy for people with autism to get a job?

It is not easy for anyone to get job autism is seen by some employers as a potential problem – others see it as a potential benefit – it would depend on the job.

This was finished on 12.03.18

Person 4: what is your understanding of autism?

Autism is a lifelong condition, it affect everyone differently, communication attached to autism.

What you think about people with autism? And how it affects people's lives?

I don't think any different of anyone with autism I just think it must be difficult because people don't understand autism properly, which must make it difficult for a person with autism.

What do I think of me and my autism?

I think you are a very outgoing person and you don't let your autism stop you doing anything once you put your mind to it.

Do I think it is easy for people with autism to get a job?

I think some people may have a struggle with the interview but I don't think this should stop them getting a job; companies should but things in place for applicants with autism.

This was finished on 12.03.18

Education

When I went to my first primary school I loved it and all the teachers where nice and my teacher assistant we were like best friends we would laugh together and joke in my own little corner in the classroom, I know I was a bit different to the other kids because when we were moving to class 6 I was doing work in year 3 to year 4 work but they were all nice and kind with me. I did a test with some random person to see if I was staying for another year after year 6 but the person said that I could go to secondary with all my friends but I was leaving all my nice teachers and the teacher assistant behind and on my last day I got very emotional because I didn't want to leave, but one day we all have to leave.

When I started my first secondary school I liked it and I was a bit nervous then things starts to change, like they moved me straight to year 7 work and they didn't really see my records or my pass, I started to cry and upset because nobody really understand autism back then like they do now, I felt like I was getting bullied by the students and more off the teachers, and teacher assistant. I used to get detention for not doing my tie but back then I didn't even know how to do a tie or my show lasses, and the kids used to pull my tie, but they was some nice teachers my favorite teacher was my drama teacher and I used to love the subject I think that's why I love acting, I used to get all my merits in my drama. I was there for 2 years and I really thought I didn't want to be here no more I used to home crying all the time in my room and I just felt giving up on life and I used to think of doing suicide so my mam got involved and got someone from the autism team to come in and get out of the school. So then I went to a special needs school with autism, but before I could go I had to get some test done to see if I had autism to get into the school and we all find out that I did have autism, it was a lovely school was there for 3 years all the teacher and teachers assistant were really nice but I felt like it was a bit too laid back so before I had another year left I left.

Whilst attending my first college I did performance art level 1, I loved it and I was cast as the main character Benvolio as well as the nurse in the Shakespearean play Romeo and Juliet. I was next cast as Mr. Snooze the main part in a comedy show. Then I went to the next level and I was so happy, yet again I got the leading cast as Jacob Marley in the Christmas carol. After that we did an old fashion show and my character was the mayor of the town. Then I did for my last show a summer show, I did a solo I sang Elton John can you feel the love and also I got a solo for dancing as well so I mixed two songs together of little mix move and the pussycat dolls don't cha, then at the end of the year we hear and see if we are moving up to the next level and I didn't because not off the performance because of the math what I think it is a bit unfair because It should be about the main course and not English and math. I was so upset because I was leaving all my close friends behind. Then I went to my second college I really didn't know what I was doing in the college because I didn't know how to draw and the teacher said that "art is not always about drawing". I felt nervous and lonely but then I made friends easy plus I loved it. I was always with the girls not with the boys as I get on better with the girls. I went to do level 3 of my first photography I loved it, I learned a lot. But yet again couldn't do the second year because of my math and English.

Now I am studying at espa college in Middlesbrough I love it here as I get along with all the amazing teachers, teachers assistant we are like one big family. It is a laid-back college and I fit in well and don't get judged. Now I am doing math and English here and feel like on the right track.

I am writing a book about autism for people to understand autism. I am passionate about music because it calms me down or if I want to be alone or if something has happened, also when I listen to some of the lyrics of the songs I can see my life in the lyrics, also I am writing songs about my life I am doing my songs writing and singing lessons with a famous person from Journey South.

Lyrics

These are my first song I have wrote and brought out on YouTube and Facebook, you can also follow my page on Facebook on diva records north east here are the lyrics to my first song.

Happy ending

V1

I had a dream about us last night
We were dancing in the sky
I was walking on cloud 9
As I stared into to your eyes

V2

we were like romeo and juliet
Cause we were never meant to be
I woke up with tears upon my pillow
Now nothing makes sense to me

Chorus

My the sun will rise again
With someone I can trust
Cause i never could trust in you
There was never a thing called Us
As Time goes by I realise
I will have have my Happy Ending

V3

You made bleed out for your love
Now Im loving someone else
He makes me makes me Feel like I can fly
The day he walked into my life

V4

And If I gave you a second chance
I''d end up in tears like i was before
Too Many heartbreaks, Too many Unanswered questions
Don't come knocking at my door

Chorus

My the sun will rise again
With someone I can trust
Cause i never could trust in you
There was never a thing called Us
As Time goes by I realise
I will have have my Happy Endin

With these lyrics and the song, it is about two people who love each other, but they can't be together so I would say something like Romeo and Juliet.

Chapter 3

Relationships

Relationships over the years have not been easy for me, I have a busy life but I haven't met the right person yet. I am happy where I am happy where I am now in my life, because I am loved by friends and family. One of my goals in my life would is to be in a loving relationship with the right person when the time is right. I know it is only a matter of time because I am a loving with a lot to give. I attend to a group called autism matters, within the group I have made some really good friends for life, I feel I can be myself and that's important to me. I feel safe with everyone and got to know more about different people with autism. I have a lot of good support with the staff, especially with one of the staff who I feel is like part of my family she is called Leanne, she's been through some tough times with me but she has seen me turn into a more positive and outgoing person. We have lots of laugh together she is also my support once a week. We do independent living we go to the gym and dance classes, every month we have a fun day out like we will go shopping or cinema.

Best friends

In autism matters I have a best friend called Natalie and we have lots of things in common we speak to each other using funny words we make up words such as shaneyanay. I can talk to Natalie about anything and she is always there for me, I am also there for her. Sometimes we have sleep overs at my house and we watch chick flicks and eat junk food and goodies. We also do our make – up and laugh with each other and I couldn't ask for a better best mate we also going to do face masks. Also my other best mate is called Dan and we always have a good time together. I can't wait to explore more things with Dan. We always tell each other everything if we are not doing something right we always tell each other and support one and other. He asked me to go away with him and his family and it was the best getaway ever. I told college I broke my toe just to sneak off as I would rather go away with my friend and his family then go to college.

On the second day of starting autism matters I went to Lightwater Valley, we went on the rides the ride was very scary. It was dark so you couldn't see anything and when we were coming down a massive hill I started to scream like a girl and then Matthew laughed and we have been best friends for 4 and a half years I have other friends, we all have, ups and downs with friends and hiccups because no friends are perfect but you need to talk to them when they do something wrong or if they upset you so they know what they are doing because you don't want to fall out, you just need to talk to each other.

The staffs are always there for their members if they need to speak to them one to one or just want to speak with one to another, I can't thank Lynne and Anna enough for their hard work and the company they provide and the hard work they do for people with autism and others spectrums. I always got along with one of the staff called Leanne. She is more of a good friend and I cannot thank her for all the support she has given me when I am at my low points.

Holiday 2018

I went to Lanzarote this year with autism matters I had a brilliant time and had lots of laugh with all the other people and the staffs they were good with everyone we all had a good time. I had a really good bond with one of the staff called Dan he really understood me I am not really get used to men with talking about myself because I sometimes feel weak and I don't want them to see me as anyone else this is why I get on with more woman then I do with men and am so happy that I could talk to him. We also had a great time in the pool using slow motion on our phones and using the jacuzzi and listening to music like shaggy wasn't me and dancing in the jacuzzi and we had people throwing cold water on us. I was still trying to be on a diet put when it comes to holiday you just eat junk food, but mainly I had pasta all week but one time I ask dan the man to make me diet coke chicken for my tea so when it was done and I was eating it the staffs were laughing while I was eating it so I said "what is so funny LOL" and then they said "nothing" but then when I finished it again dan the man said "did you enjoy your food" and I said "yes" thanks dan then he had a secret to tell me he said to me "I didn't use diet coke he used full fat coke". So the next day without him seeing I pushed him into the pool and I loved it. On the full last day we went to this place I can't remember the place new went to but apparently vogue magazine goes there to take pictures because it was such a beautiful place. I really got on with one of the other staff called Howard we don't really talk as much as I do with the other staff but since I've been on holiday with him I see us having a real good bond and I loved pushing him into the pool, me and Lynee are like two gossip girl we love chatting about make-up and girly talks and yet again she is always there for everyone.

Person 5: what is your understanding of autism?

My understanding is that the brain is wired differently and makes them see things in a different light of from another perspective.

What you think about people with autism? And how it affects people's lives?

I don't think anything in particular, I think it is a different way of living; however I know they have very different struggles I think it affects people in different ways as there is different levels of autism.

What do I think of me and my autism?

I think it makes you unique, and who you are.

Do I think it is easy for people with autism to get a job?

Employers are not allowed to discriminate against, however I think sometimes they may be over cautions.

This was finished on 12.03.18

Person 6: what is your understanding of autism?

Autism is a lifelong neuro developmental condition it can affect about to communicate effectually and can restrict behaviors. I have a lot of training and understand more than the general propulsions.

What you think about people with autism? And how it affects people's lives?

Autism should not define you a step you doing anything. It affects people in different ways. Some people struggle with it more than others.

What do I think of me and my autism?

You don't let your autism stop you from attempting anything you embrace it and live life to the fullest.

Do I think it is easy for people with autism to get a job?

I think it can be very difficult, as it does not often understand but employers, and can lead to judgement capability sells can go unnoticed.

This was finished on 12.03.18

Person 7: what is your understanding of autism?

Autism is a lifelong condition. It affects people with their communication skills.

What you think about people with autism? And how it affects people's lives?

I think autism affects people in different ways. It does affects people's lives but with lots of encouragement you can achieve what you want in life.

What do you think of me and my autism?

I think you are an inspiration to other people with autism. You don't let anything hold you back.

Do you think it is easy for people with autism to get a job?

I think it is harder for people with autism to get a job but not impossible. Companies just need to know more aware and understanding towards autism.

This was finished on 12.03.18

Chapter 4

Person 8: what is your understanding of autism?

Autism is a lifelong condition I think life could be very difficult for a person with autism as sometimes has many different condition attached with autism.

What you think about people with autism? And how it affects people's lives?

I don't think of a person with autism any different to any other person. I just think they need a little more help/support to achieve their goals. Autism affects people's lives in much different way's social/relationship behavioral.

What do you think of me and my autism?

I think you are a very unique person and your autism doesn't seem to affect you, and your personality always makes me smile, but you are a drama queen.

Do you think it is easy for people with autism to get a job?

I don't think having autism should make a different in getting a job, but it may be harder for them.

This was finished on 12.03.18

Person 9: what is your understanding of autism?

I have a very good knowledge of autism and other related conditions.

What you think about people with autism? And how it affects people's lives?

People with autism are very intelligent and sometimes can be left out of things. Society is the thing that needs to change to accept people with autism. People with autism can do anything they can put their mind too with support or without.

What do you think of me and my autism?

You are a very friendly intelligent person and have a good sense of humor works hard.

Do you think it is easy for people with autism to get a job?

Yes and no it is down to each individual person and how much determination you want a job.

This was finished on 13.03.18

Person 10: what is your understanding of autism?

Autism is a disability development that affects how a person communicates and relates to a people around them. It is commonly known as autism spectrum disorder (ASD). Children and adults with autism have difficulties with social interaction in everyday life.

Autism is a complex neurodevelopmental condition that impairs social interaction and language development and communication skills; combined with rigid and repetitive behavior. Some children and adults with autism may have trouble communicating. They have difficulties understanding what other people think and feel.

In children with ASD, the symptoms are present before three years of age, although a diagnosis can be made at any time during their life.

How can autism affect people's lives?

Some people with autism are able to live relatively independent lives, but others may have accompanying learning disabilities and need a lifetime of specialist support.

People with autism may have difficulties with social interaction and could be unaware of what is socially appropriate. They may find chatting or small talk difficult and may not be able to socialize very much. They may appear uninterested in and find it extremely difficult to develop friendships and struggle mixing with people.

Those affected may be able to speak or may they be nonverbal. There may also be difficulties understanding gestures, body language, facial expressions and tone of voice, making it difficult to judge or understanding the reactions of those they are talking to or to empathies with people's feelings. As a result, they may unintentionally appear insensitive or rude to others. They may also take other people's comments literally and misunderstanding what people say.

What do I think of bob and his autism?

I have known bob for many years now, having been his teaching assistant at school and his support worker, which I was for a number of years. Although bob did need quite a lot of support during academic lessons he was pretty independent when it came to lessons like art, food tech and most of all music. It was his love of music that brought us to work together a lot during his schools years. Especially as I was the choir and theatre co-ordinator. He particularly enjoyed singing and was always eager to do solo performances in school events which gave him a lot of the confidence he has today.

He was always happy go lucky and fun to be around. He loved nothing more than a good chat about soaps, school, his family and friends he always coped extremely well with his autism never allowing it to stop him fulfilling things that he wanted to achieve. With the support of his amazing family bob completed his school years going onto.

Performing arts at college where he took part in some brilliant shows and concerts often having a singing and speaking part which he coped with brilliantly. He then went onto art college and then onto following his dream which is where he is now. I can only say how extremely proud I am to know bob and was lucky enough to be apart of his life growing up. I wish him all the very best for his future and everything he does.

Do you think it is easy for people with autism to get a job and follow their dreams?

Autism affects so many people in so many different ways. Being an adult on the autistic spectrum can be wonderful and challenging! I personality think from experience that people on the autism spectrum can go on to achieve their dreams. I have worked with children who have gained amazing qualifications, obtained their dreams job or even started a family of their own.

This was finished on 08.10.18

Person 11: what is your understanding?

People with autism see the world through a different perspective they find social skills very difficult and struggle to understand emotions

How can autism affect people's lifes?

Autistic people find social skills very difficult. The find it hard to read emotions and find normal everyday things hard. They like routine and when that changes they get very stressed and emotional.

What do I think of bob and his autism.

Bobby was definitely a character. I felt bobby was very funny and he made me laugh. He was such a drama queen and was always in trouble for kissing the girls. He never much liked doing any work and used to cry a lot when asked to do it. He was lovely though and I enjoyed working with him very much.

Do you think it is easy for people with autism to get a job and follow their dreams?

Yes. As more people understand autism it is easier for work places to accept them. Sometimes it is good for them to volunteer to help them with social skills.

Person 12: So what is your understanding of autism?

My understanding of autism it is affects people in lots of different ways. I don't think it is something that affects 2 people in the same way. It doesn't always affect people negatively it sometimes comes with things where people are creative, maybe people can solve problems whereas someone who doesn't have autism couldn't it allows people to think differently. It does come with its challenges and people with autism have issues sometimes around relationships or it might be something to do with the world around us like sounds or light that type of thing. It affects a lot of people in a lot of different ways.

How can autism affect people different ways?

The person with autism I suppose it can affect them in lots of ways in all areas in their life. They might need a bit extra support in certain areas that they are affected more by. It might be with accessing social events or it might be with having a full-time job. They might just need a bit of help and support and whether that's a different timetable or whether that is been shown how to do something rather then told how to do something. It can affect people in lots of different ways but it's about understanding the person with autism and their unique needs they have got.

What do you think of me and my autism?

I think your absolutely brilliant I think you're a laugh a minute I think you always have a funny story to tell, you have always got a new hair colour always got a new piercing in your ear. With you bobby you very kind and caring person you make friends quite easy everyone seems to like you, you are the life and soul of every party. I think you will be able to tell me more than I can, I think the way autism affects you, maybe people don't see it on the surface with you maybe I wouldn't be able to tell if you were having a bad day. You don't present any sort of any mood where I would be able to tell oh bobby is having a bad day, you sort of keep it inside yourself, I think you release it in different ways maybe one to one with Leanne, or maybe going to the gym or listening to music or singing. I think it affects you maybe deeper down than it does other people. Other people are more on the surface, does that make sense?

Do you think it should be easier for people with autism to work or have a career in what they want to do?

Yes absolutely, I think in terms of opportunities I think there are more opportunities nowadays. but I think there needs to be more understanding of the support someone needs with autism in the work places don't have the awareness or aren't structured around different people with different need. I think if people are more aware than they can, put things in place and as far as opportunities go, if you're right for the job regardless of physical abilities, your age, your gender or if you have autism the job should be there for you. I do think things are positively changing I think there are opportunities out there and there is more understanding but there is still a long way to go.

Person 13:

My understanding of autism is that it affect individuals on the autistic spectrum in different ways. I believe that autistic people view the world differently.

Autism can make life challenging for individuals as not everyone is adequately equipped to deal will the needs of autistic people, due to lack of experience or misinformation.

I think that autism has not held you back in your life, and it has helped you to become a sensitive, creative person.

I strongly believe in equality and diversity and equal opportunities for everyone.

The fun times for me were when you were working on your essay "The lady of Shalott" and also "Coco Chanel", when we would discuss certain aspects of the stories and you would relate them to dramas you'd seen on the tele or pop stars lives. Spending time doing photography was great with you especially in the darkroom.

The thing I found funniest was when you did a lot of quirk on the computer and then couldn't remember where you'd saved it, then we would have to do all of the work again, or I would, normally during my lunch break.

Person 14: So what is your understanding of autism?

Autism is a lifelong developmental disability that affects how people perceive the world and interact and communicate with others. Autistic people see, hear and feel the world differently to other people. If you are autistic, you are autistic for life; autism is not an illness or disease and cannot be 'cured'. Autism is a spectrum condition. All autistic people share certain difficulties, but being autistic will affect them in different ways. People with autism may also experience over – or under – sensitivity to sounds, touch, tastes, smells, lights or colours.

How can autism affect people different ways?

Some people with autism are able to live relatively independent lives, but others may have accompanying learning disabilities and need a lifetime of specialist support.

Do you think it should be easier for people with autism to work or have a career in what they want to do?

Yes I strongly agree that people with autism should find it easier to find employment and be well supported throughout people who has autism make amazing employee's and need to be given much more support to find work and business need to give people with autism much more opportunity to do so.

What do you think of me and my autism?

You're just amazing! You support your friends who have autism, make people, laugh brightens everyone's day and you are one of the nicest people I know, I'm so glad we met and my son has you as his friend. He loves seeing you and so do we don't EVER CHANGE X. everyone adores you bobby. You so funny everyone needs a bobby in their life.

Person 15: So what is your understanding of autism?

For me autism is different for each person. So a diagnosis of autism means you have difficulty with commutating with understanding social situations and difficulties with imagination sometimes or repetitive thoughts.

How can autism affect people different ways?

It can impact on people's lifes in lots of ways. If someone with autism has sensory issues, then just doing everyday things like going out into the sunshine, or wearing certain clothes can be really difficult for them, but also if you have a lack of understanding and communication then communicating in the world is really difficult so if they don't like been around people then that can be a really difficult situation because it can be a really social world.

What do you think of me with autism and how it affects my life?

Autism affects people in lots of different ways. Not everyone is going to be the same and how it affects them. I think with you because your such high functioning in lots of ways you have really good communication and social and language skills, that lots of people would not see your autism initially when they get to know you as a person then you kind of see how literal you take things, so that if someone tells you something you believe them and take things literally. You trust everyone around you and don't know when people are lying to you.

Person 16: So what is your understanding of autism?

It affects people in different ways, some can talk some can't some have problems in social situations and some don't. some have to have specific instructions what to do and have to speak to people in certain ways, that's how I see it.

What do you think of me with autism and how it affects my life?

Your one of my best friends, you drive me absolutely crazy sometimes but that's just because people with autism don't always get along because the autism fight each other. Something that affects you doesn't affect me vies versa. So sometimes my jokes might not be your kind of humour and it can cause us to fall out. Sometimes your humour does my head in and I think you're a bit silly, but there you are.

Do you think it should be easier for people with autism to work?

No, it's not easy as people think it is, it depends on how the people you work for treat you. If you get the proper training the proper help then yeah, but it's not easy as you think.

How does autism affect people's lifes, so how does autism affect your life?

It tricky to know what people without autism are thinking, you can't always tell if they are telling jokes, you can't always understand what they mean. Sometimes you can misinterpret what they mean it can cause problems causes stress in your family life. Your parents have taught you to do things a certain way but you can't always do it that way cause you can't always understand what to do. It's hard to make friends it's hard to make relationships, friends + boyfriends + girlfriends type of thing, but as long as you have friends and stuff it's alright but it is really hard to do.

What do you think about autism matters?

I haven't been to autism matters that long. I didn't get diagnosed till i was 17 – 18 years old. I have not had the help as much as other people without autism matters I wouldn't be half the person i am today, I wouldn't have as many friends, I wouldn't understand as much, I wouldn't of met you and let's be honest that would probably of been better, but you are one of my best friends like I said and I wouldn't have life now without that, best friends and that.

Chapter 5

Person 17: Some people seem to think you can outgrow autism and I want to make it clear. You never outgrow it, autism is a lifelong condition you are born with so even if you go traveling or work you still have autism. Your just achieving things in your life. Autism just not prevent you from having a healthy social life and you should not be penalized for it. For it. Sometimes it's a rigorous. Process to get what you're entitled to and it can put some genuine people off.

How does autism affect you?

Mainly I would say autism is kind of myself is a part of me and I wouldn't want to change that it kind of defines who I am I also have with that O.C.D. which is O.C.D. I would say that is the thing that I would need to combat, like fight against so I would say that if someone would take my autism away I would like someone to take away the O.C.D. that's my general answer.

Do you think it's easy for people with autism to work?

You definitely have strengths that can be put forward. Everybody is so different on the autistic spectrum which depends on the individual I'd say general traits are hard working methodical, organized things like that, but sometimes they can struggle. Obviously with social interaction which can make it difficult to function in the work place. In addition the sensory issues they have can make it difficult to function in a working environment such as bright lights, loud noises and papers rustling things like that.

What is your understanding of autism?

What do I know about autism, from what I know, lifelong developmental disability that affects the away in which a person see the world, so to do with the way that the neurons in the brain form and its means that it's difficult for people with autism to pick up on social skills, there is also a triad of impairments I can't remember what they are.

Person 18:

What is your understanding of autism?

I think that every person with autism is different, no 2 people with autism are the same. That everyone with autism will have difficulty in the same areas. Autism is a spectrum, so there are some people with autism, what would you call high function. People who are very intelligent but still have the same difficulties and there are other people with autism who have learning difficulties and they might not have any language. Probably the most people I work with in this place the biggest struggles for them, that are associated with autism is they struggle to understand people, so communication is quite a big one. Communication doesn't just mean what people say it's how they say it. Understanding peoples body language, understanding how their behavior might make other people feel, so it really is an invisible disability really in a nut shell but there is a lot more I can add. Same difficulties with the way their brain works, someone on reception has autism, he comes here and he has support.

How can autism effects people's lifes?

I guess a lot of people I know with autism have got some mental health problems so they can feel really anxious or maybe quite depressed, because they want to live a normal life, they want to live a full life but sometimes because of other people, because other people don't understand what their needs are they struggle to do that. It can affect your life in lots of ways I guess obviously it can affect your relationships, building friendships with people you can trust, understanding people and safe relationships. Like I said it's a big one for you isn't it. I think it's probably, I read somewhere once having autism is like going to a foreign country and been able to say I can speak/5 words in French then going to France and been lost everything gets lost so a lot of people with autism have sensory problems so they struggle when they take in lots of information so they feel on edge all of the time. They feel quite stressed all the time. The information that is important that they need to take in they miss out on because they have too much information in their heads. It's almost liked a computer, overheating so they maybe need that time to be by themselves and sort their head out and get everything straight. When they get a bit, older relationships change it might be romantic relationships and they may not understand what they mean because not everyone says what they mean. People sometimes give you a wink, their body language might communicate more also I think it's probably quite a confusing world for people to live in, they might find it overwhelming.

What do you think about me with autism & how I cope?

I think that you cope, some people with autism can be quite & quite shy and quite anxious and maybe you are quite anxious but I think you might mask it sometimes with your behavior, you can be a it of a joker and it always probably depends for you I think bobby on what environment you're in, so if you comfortable with somebody like you are a bit of a joker. Your passionate about everything you do, so you have special interests like you used to do drama didn't you. You were really interested in that but I think you don't mind me saying I think your vulnerable with relationships you've always wanted to have certain relationships, you struggle to understand. You always think that because the way you think is the way the everybody else thinks it's not the case. Sometimes I think you can get yourself into difficult situations because you don't pick up on what people mean just because someone says it doesn't mean. I think I don't know are you a socialable person, I don't know, yeah probably, if you're comfortable with the people if your comfortable I think you are. I think you have found things that you have been really passionate about and interested in which a lot of people with autism do and sometimes can come a bit obsessed. I think you are lovely to work with I will never forget you.

Do you think it is easy for people with autism to work or be who thy want to be?

Not always, I think it's about other people understanding really, I think if you have got support in the work place and other people understand what the difficulties are then it might be easier, but again I think because it is an invisible disability and it's not obvious that you have got a disability, that it's not until you start to work and somebody asks you to do something and you don't understand what they want you to do, but then you might find it hard to ask for the help and keep all the information in your head in the right order, I think that were the difficulties are. I think it's difficult for anyone with autism sometimes to work even if they are super intelligent because they have still got the problems that there are born with.

Person 19:

What is your understanding of autism?

For me autism is different for each person. So, a diagnosis of autism means you have difficulty with communicating with understanding social situations and difficulties with imagination sometimes or repetitive thoughts.

How can autism affect people's autism?

It can impact people's lives in lots of ways. If someone with autism has sensory issues, then just doing everyday things like going out into the sunshine, or wearing certain clothes can be really difficult for them, but also if you have a lack of understanding and communication then communicating in the world is really difficult so if they don't like being around people then that can be a really difficult situation because it can be a really social world.

What do you think of me with autism and how it affects my life?

Autism affects people in lots of different ways. Not everyone is going to be the same and how it affects them. I think with you because your such high functioning in lots of ways you have really good communication and social and language skills, that lots of people would not see your autism initially when they get to know you as a person then you kind of see how literal you take things, so that if someone tells you something you believe them and take things literally. You trust everyone around you and don't know when people are lying.

Person 20:

What is your understanding of autism?

My understanding of autism is people think, they see people with autism and think oh he's weird or she's weird, but who's to say they are weird or we are weird. Doesn't means to say that the way people think with autism is right or whether it's wrong, it how it's perceived, they can be a bit strange and some people think to be autistic they like things in the same place autism, the autism spectrum comes from the floor to the top and it varies so much and I know that every person with autism is completely different and what they tell you is the truth and what they tell you sometimes it's not what you want to hear. They don't understand it's not what you want to hear but it is the truth.

What do you think about me with autism and how it affects my life?

Well when you were in the school, I didn't sort of think of you of having autism and I just used to think you were a lovely outgoing boy, you were really outgoing you were pleasant and you would say what you're thinking you would say what you think and you were always laughing and giggling and you enjoyed life. You always enjoyed life and you weren't like some people with autism who like to be secluded on their own. You weren't in that category you like to be with friends and I thought you were really good at socializing. You socialize and you could make friends with anybody male, females, old, young, staff and student made no difference to you, who they were, what age and it was lovely to see that you could do that and you had some good banter, really good banter. When you were moving to Beverley I thought it was a sad day, it was a sad thing cos I thought you were coping with mainstream. Been in mainstream, you didn't stand out as anything. You were, to me just average Jo Bloggs. I thought you were coping well in mainstream. To me you problem wasn't your autism it was your learning. It was your learning you found difficult not coping with your autism. When you get to year 9 it's your sexuality joins in and your hormones are well over the place and when your autistic your feelings are all over the place and quite difficult. Autism is like a jigsaw and you can't put the pieces together, what's missing what's wrong somethings different and when you go through puberty it is difficult and I do think it is harder for someone with autism to go through puberty rather than someone without autism. Even children with learning disabilities can tend not to cope with it very well and especially girls because they have ladies problems and they can't deal with it.

Do you think it is easy for people with autism to work or get what they want in life?

The advantage of having autism is your focused on what you want to do and you make it your goal. Like the boy I know and work with he is fixated on engineering, on how things work and because he fixates on it he has become quite expert on it, so because you have got that focus and you can put everything into it I think whatever you want to achieve you can do it. Anything you want to do you set that goal, put your mind to it you can do it.

How does autism affect people?

We have a young boy who comes here and he is struggling at the minute. It's difficult for him when things are going on, like places like corridors when they are busy. We have another boy who can't bear to be touched you are not allowed to run but because he can't bear to be touched he is always running. it can be difficult in such a big school like this if you are on the autistic spectrum, because of the noise the business of the place, there are always changes going on, you have got the changing of lessons, the changing of teachers and teacher who are going to be off so you need cover. Everyday we take things for granted that someone with autism there is so many change, in a short period of time it can difficult. My heart goes out to anyone with autism who I know is struggling, you can see it in their face. To get though everyday life it's a struggle.

Person 21:

Why did you thought I had autism?

I noticed very early on that something was not right with my son he was not making is normal milestones for his age , his speech was very delayed and his sitting up and walking his communication skills were very delayed also so it was clear to me that they was something going on he was very quiet and sleeper a lot also

So mam what do you think of my first primary school?

I thought the school was a really good school, you were there for a little while but Mr. Dunn was the head teacher at the time decided that he thought that you weren't going to cope with the school. That it was going to be too difficult and that you would need a more specialized school, so we decided that you would go to your second primary school which you were very happy with. You came on really well in the school. You were there for a few years and it was the right place for you, it taught you so many things and you came on leaps and bounds, it was really good. But the school started to introduce children with behavioral problems, and I had to make a decision because you didn't really have behavioral problems you had a learning disabilities and autism so I didn't want you mixing with people with behavioral problems, so I made the decision to take you out of the school and to put you back into your first primary school again because I thought that it would be too much for you and I didn't want you picking up on the children with the bad behavioral problems, it was a real shame because up until the school had been very good.

What is the difference between ADHD and autism?

There isn't a difference between ADHD and autism these are two totally different conditions although it is quite common to find that someone with ADHD could be found to be on the autistic spectrum.

What did you think of my second primary school?

The school was a very good school for my son as it first off all was safe and they understand the way that people with autism should be taught unlike a mainstream school I had to take my son out of mainstream school as he was not progressing the way he should have been and his interaction was also very different.

What did you think of the second time that I went to my first primary school again?

For the second time again it wasn't right place for you because they didn't have a unit there at the point. If they had of had a unit it would have been a very different story and I think you would have been ok there but they didn't have it and you needed full 1:1 support and the school were not able to support you in that way so it wasn't going to be the right place.

What did you think of my first secondary school?

Initially I thought the school was going to be really good but I was really disappointed, I didn't think that they understood children with a learning disability, I thought a lot of teachers were very abrupt and I knew that it wasn't the right place because your behavior, just went off the scale and I knew I needed to get you diagnosed to get you out of there, because it defiantly wasn't the right place for you.

How old was I when I got diagnosed?

I think you were about 12 and it was Dr Helen pears who diagnosed you, although I knew that you already had autism. I was aware of that, but we needed an official diagnosis & she came and worked for many months with you and she actually give you the diagnosis if autism & having a learning disability.

What did you think of the second secondary school I went to?

I liked the school, it was a bit of a culture shock because they were children with different severities, so although I knew it was a safe place for you and the majority of the time you were very happy there, and within your class mainly the children were on the same spec as you but it was a little bit hard because there was different children with different degrees of autism, so I did find it quite hard but I could see that you were happy there and that you were thriving there and you were also there for a few years, so yeah it was the right place for you.

What did you think of the first college I went to?

The college, it was a big step and a big decision for you to make, you made the decision to come out of the school & I think it was the right decision at the time. But the college was always going to be a challenge even though you were happy & it was a lovely college & the work you did you really enjoyed, you did some really good performances and you were really happy there and also very vulnerable there and got yourself into a couple of little hiccups, or shall we say big hiccups! and it was the same in the other college as well.

What did you think of the second college I went to?

Again the same as the first college it was a lovely college and you did enjoy it. You were up and down with the course you chose but again you were very vulnerable with the other people in there. You were very easily lead and it wasn't a safe haven like the other colleges had been. It was a bit difficult because even though you strived to be what we say normal you did have your autism and the teachers were very supportive and it's a really nice college and you did really well and the teachers said you should be so proud because the 2 years you spent there you gained a lot of awards when it came to the 3rd year it became the same as the first college it just got too academic, but it was a learning process for you and I think it was still good, although you were very vulnerable within side the college.

What did you think of the other day center I went to?

You didn't spend a lot of time at the place it was maybe just one day a week or two days a week and you did enjoy it, it was a lovely place and they were always very accommodating to what you wanted to do. I was very happy with the place.

What do you think of my first year of my 3rd college?

Your first year and second year I think it was the right place for you although you found it a little bit difficult because you felt like you took a step back, on another angle you were learning and thriving and you were in a safe place with people of similar abilities and I think you liked the staff. The staff are like your friends and I think you like that aspect of it. You grumble sometimes that that they were a bit laid back on the other hand if it had not been to laid back and they had pushed you more than you could deal with you, you would have grumbled about that. I think the college has been the perfect place for you. It helped you to mature a lot.

What do you think about me writing a book?

Well I'm very proud of you, I think that it's a big challenge for you writing a book and with the help that you getting I'm very grateful so for all the people that care helping you. I think it's a wonderful thing and when people do read it I think they will get a lot out of it and they will see your journey and life so far.

What do you think of me writing my own songs?

I think that' wonderful Bobby writing your own songs, I think the last one you have written is absolutely fantastic and I think it good because you love that and get a lot of enjoyment and happiness form that I think it's good. I'm very proud of you.

Person 22:

What is your understanding of autism?

My understand of autism is that it's a condition that affects people's social skills and their ability to communicate with other people. It affects their behavior and day to day life really.

How can autism affect people's life?

It affects their life because obviously they struggle communicating, they struggle to make friendships they struggle socially, they struggle to mix with their peer group they struggle to communicate with everyone really even doctors or people in shops. Everybody struggles with different aspects because obviously people autism it affects people different it can affect their day to day life.

What do you think of me with autism and how it affects my life?

Your autism makes you who you are, you know like, I could not imagine you any different you are gorgeous, funny loving caring a diva like all the time, but I also see how it affects you with your emotions and how you struggle to read other people's emotions and struggle to deal with your own emotions and interpret them but that just makes you who you are. You are just loveable and friendly to be around.

Do you think it should be easier for people with autism to work and have a career?

I definitely think they should be more opportunities for people with autism to work and for people to show what skills they have because obviously people with autism their attention to detail and their ability to follow a task from end to end and their time keeping their honesty there all brilliant skulls to take into a work place and I think if people have more understanding of that they would see the benefits that someone with autism could bring to the work place definitely.

Person 23:

What was your first experience of autism?

My son was diagnosed at 3 years old before that I didn't know what autism was when he was diagnosed, I decided to find out as much as possible about it in order to help him in his life. I would make sure I taught him in my own way even potty training. I would decide to teach him three things each week which was hard as a single mum. One of the hardest things was when my son would shut himself away in his bedroom as he would like his own company. When he was two, he would only eat rice pudding even for his Christmas dinner.

How long have you worked at this place and do you enjoy it?

I've worked at this place for two years I really enjoy it because must days I go away thinking I have made a difference to people's lives. Of course there are bad days but most of the time it is very fulfilling. I love the vanity and developing relationship with the students.

How did your son cope with his autism?

When he was old enough to release the implications of autism he was worried but learned to adapt to situations he found socializing difficult even going out for family meals he wouldn't talk. It was therefore a process of trying to improve. He went to university at Sunderland which was a big step because of living on his own so I had to teach him certain skills like cooking other thing, like washing were a problem but he had to overcome these problems and find a solution. He then had the opportuning to go to china for 10 months. This involved me preparing him to live half way round the world. I was nervous but knew it was the opportunity of a lifetime. I had to prepare him for all the injection he would new for the trip which was difficult as he hated needles. I went with him the first time then encouraged him to go on his own. He then felt ok and got the confidence to go on his own. I always say to my son don't ever let autism hold you back, don't use it as an excuse, always aim high. He was learnt to drive and has a very full orchestra. He goes to the gym and plays golf. He is currently looking for a job and I know he will always be great at whatever he does.

Person 24:

What is your understanding of autism?

Autism is a lifelong disability which benefits from a different way of learning. A person with autism may look at things in a different way to others and may find it difficult to communicate.

What do you think about people with autism and how it affects peoples life?

I think people with autism are very brave to overcome some of their difficulty's as some people do not understand how difficult certain things may feel to a person with autism. I think it takes a lot of hard determination to get though something you are very anxious about. Some people don't understand how hard is for someone with autism to do something they struggle with and think that because they are comfortable with it is everyone is.

What do you think of me and my autism?

Bobby, I think you are amazing you try your hardest at what you (your book) you're a kind person who cares for others as well as yourself. You get on with everyone and are always happy unless you don't get your own way haha. I think you deal with your autism so well and are growing as a person.

Do you think it is easy for people with autism to work?

I don't think it is easy for anyone to get a job and it can knock your confidence if you don't get a job you want so I think it is very possible for people with autism to work it may be hard at times with some of a person's struggles and hard top deal with some of the knock backs jobs can bring but with the right help it would be very good for them and enjoyable.

This was finished on 25.06.19

Couple months ago, I was getting ready putting my make up on and singing away in the bathroom, when I was finished I tried to open the door but it wouldn't open, then all I heard was my mam's partner giggling outside the door he was saying hahaha, I knew by then he was playing a trick on me I found it funny but I only had ten minutes till I went out with autism matters, so I was screaming open the door NOW, he keep on giggling and I was laughing as well, luckily I had my phone to ring my mam because she was in the park with my sister and her dogs and all I heard was them laughing through the phone, so I started laughing again, so my mam rang him up to let me out so then he did, I found out he kept the door shut by tying my mams dressing gown rope to the bathroom door handle to the other door handle. This is our humor in the house.

America

Sunday, the day before I went to America I was a model for eyelash lift. I went to the cinema with my friend Dan to watch end game marvel. It was on for 3 and half hours, everyone was crying except me. When it finished we went to Dan's flat to get his holiday things, and he left his keys and stuff with his staff. We went to mine house and had pizza and gin with lemonade, we were excited. We only had a couple of hours sleep as we had to be up for. My sister picked us up she flew through the traffic as we had to be there for 5am at tees barrage. Me, Matthew and Dan sat together on the bus messing around, I had some strawberry Bon Bon's by Bobby's and then a girl laughed and start calling me bobby bon – bon and everyone laughed. We got to the airport in 2 and a half later we went through checkout and it was fine. We then went to burger king our orders were wrong but we kept calm. Me, Matthew and Dan went to the toilet but then got lost on the way back, but then went the right way and meet up with the rest of the gang. We got on the plane through fast track while we were going through fast track there were people talking about us, because for getting the fast tracked, one of the staff explained why we got the fast track. We all got on the plane ok but I had a panic attack when we took off. The Women next to me give me a boiled sweet. I was doing my script on the plane and speaking to the woman who give me the sweet, she was asking who I came on holiday with I told her Autism Matters. She was telling me she thinks her grandson may have autism. I got myself some new perfume. We had some turbulence I was screaming, because we dropped a couple of feet. The food wasn't nice on the plane, we landed in America. We then hired a minibus, we got to the villa and got our room's I went into my friend room Joanne "I said I like your room can I have it!" and she said "yes". We all went out for our tea, I was not keen on the food it was fatty and oily. We then went shopping for our own food and drinks. I got cherry Smirnoff vodka then I got some cherry Fanta to go with it. On the Saturday I went to swim with the dolphins we had a lagoon it was a dream come true. We also got to kiss them and stroke them, we went snorkelling some members were braver than me and Matthew every time we got in the pool it was getting colder and colder we were just laughing at each other. We finally got in the water we swam with the fish and stingrays, if a stingray came past you could stroke it. I went into an area in the pool and thought I could go under but hit my head on the glass Anna and Matthew were laughing, and then we just chilled in our private area. When we were waiting for the dolphins we were waiting for breakfast and I was messing around with an orange peel. Before we got to the entrance of discovery cove, a woman who worked there was holding a sloth we could touch it. On the same night I heard Matthew and Dan talking about watching the new episode of games of thrones so I came up with a plan and I said, I am not a big fan of games of thorns but because you are my two best friends I will make I deal with Matthew. If he came with me to see the curse of Llorna I would watch one episode of game of thorns, so we made a deal and shook on it. On that night while everyone was in bed me, Matthew, Dan and Lynne stayed up to watch game of thorns on Dan's fire stick. While we were watching it, it was buffering all the time Matthew was getting wound up, Matthew always wind me up so I came up with a plan to wind him up, when I seen Matthew getting wound up I started eating popcorn to wind him up more. Lynne started laughing. The next day we went to volcano bay and got an $800 private area. I felt like beonce with my big glasses on. Me Anna Mathew and Dan went on our first water ride, me and Mathew were at the back I screamed like a girl and everyone laughed at me.

Then we went on agene this time with lynee. Mathew Dan and Anna were secretly recording and put it in Facebook. On the night time we were all playing cards "against humanity "and it was funny to play with Anna and Lynne.

The next day we went to the theme park I went on the harry potter ride, and screamed my head off as I did on most of the rides. We went to a place called voodoo donuts the donut was huge, outside the place there was a voodoo donut chair we all got a photo took on the chair. I got a photo took of the universal globe. We went to Epcot. On a different day we went to a different theme park I went on.

The mummy ride – on the mummy ride I was very anxious but I was very proud of myself for trying a new ride, the first time I went with Lynne, Matthew and Dan were in front, Matthew turned around ask me if I was ok and laughing, and I said "shut up". There was warning sign saying the ride goes backwards, Matthew and Dan seen and didn't warn me and were laughing at me. When the ride was going it was dark and I was holding onto Lynne very tight, I said does this ride go backwards, she said no. the ride stopped at a dead-end and then went backwards, Lynne was laughing because I was screaming.

Pirates of Caribbean water ride – I was sat next to Matthew, Lynne and Dan, it was very dark the ride and I don't really like water rides I ask Lynne if there were any big hills she said "no". I could feel us going and Matthew and lynee were laughing because they knew what was going to happen it went down really fast I screamed and got soaked.

On the Friday we went to the theme park we all went to see frozen show at the end there was fake snow falling. Some of us went to see the muppet show me and Matthew were board hoping for it to end, at the end there was a bubble machine.

On our last day we went to the shops before going to the airport. I got a shiny rose gold glitter hat I thought I'm buying that it suits me. Then me and Matthew went into a marvel shop and got our photo as a super hero. I was black widow and Matthew was captain America. Outside the Lego shop there was people getting in a car that drives on top of water. On the way back home I sat with Matthew and had another panic attack, I was holding Matthew's arm tight and he was laughing at me.

A couple of week later I went to the cinema to see the curse of lanorna at that time Matthew dad dropped me off. Matthew got the tickets, he laughed because we were the only two for that film and the whole screen, 15 mins in the film I went to the toilet. When I came back I hid behind the wall trying to scare Matthew. I jumped and screamed because the scary part came on, we were jumping when the scary parts came on.

My birthday 2018 my sister has surprised me with a two hour singing lesson. The day before my singing lesson I went to group and Lynne and Leanne said to me "I'm sure one of the brothers from journey south lives there" and I said "No why would he live there he will be rich by now". On the day of my singing lesson my brother took me to his house and I said "wow this is a big house" then he opened the door and he was a very nice man.

I looked around his house and I said "wow massive studio" and looked around and I said "wow you have a lot of guitars in your house" so then I had the balls to ask him "are you one of the brothers from journey south?" and he said "well yes I am" and in my head I was saying "well I am not singing in front of you" so I decided to ask him if it was ok if I write my own songs will he sing my songs and he said "yes no problem" and ever since I have been working with him co-writing my songs for around 14 months now. I had brought out 5 songs with my songs I want to help out people in bad relationships to escape bad relationships I have wrote a song about the Manchester bombing and I have also written songs about mental illness. I write the songs sometimes Carl will edit them Carl also does the music and produces the song, he also brings in other singers to sing my songs.

If you would like to contact me to give me an opportunity to be a songwriter please can you contact me on my Facebook page or Instagram page under the name diva records north east if you would like to have an interview with me about my music and my book please contact me again on the same page. I would like to have interviews and I would love to work on radio stations such as capital, TFM or BBC tees.

Thank you

This is the first song I have ever done

Happy ending

V1
I had a dream about us last night
We were dancing in the sky
I was walking on cloud 9
As I stared into to your eyes

V2
we were like romeo and juliet
Cause we were never meant to be
I woke up with tears upon my pillow
Now nothing makes sense to me

Chorus

My sun will rise again
With someone I can trust
Cause i never could trust in you
There was never a thing called Us
As Time goes by I realise
I will have my Happy Ending

V3
You made me bleed out for your love
Now Im loving someone else
He makes me Feel like I can fly
The day he walked into my life

V4

And If I gave you a second chance
I''d end up in tears like i was before
Too Many heartbreaks, Too many Unanswered questions
Don't come knocking at my door

Chorus

My sun will rise again
With someone I can trust
Cause i never could trust in you
There was never a thing called Us
As Time goes by I realise
I will have my Happy Endin

This song is about two people who can't be together so it's a bit like Romeo and Juliet.
This finished on 19/06/18
Bobby latheron

This is my second one
NOBODY KNOWS LYRICS

Verse 1

Nobody know when i cry at
night i was thinking about me
nobody knows that i wake up
somedays

wishing i was gone then
an angel came to me and
said you amazed me with
your strength

you make it through this
dont you worry about a thing
be happy with the skin you leaving
in

Chorus

Nobody knows how i really
feel these cuts even close
to healing how can I
show all i can be
to many people made my
life a misery nobody knows

Verse 2

I thought i was someone that
was broken that i needed
fixing i had to go
to hell and back to find

what i was missing with this

words i clanged my soul
i just wanted to let u
know this storm will pass
this pain cant last the
sun will help me to heal

Chorus

Nobody knows how i really
feel these cuts even close
to healing how can I
show all i can be
when to many people made
my life a misery nobody knows

Bridge

I was given another chance
another shot at happiness I
thought you were the one
how could i be so wrong
now im

shattered to pieces like broken
its like the wind and
the trees were saying to
me go find yourself before
you fall again before putting someone
else in your life

Chorus

Nobody knows how i really
feel these scars even close
to healing how can I
show how i really feel
when too many people made
my life a misery nobody knows

This song is about mental illness nobody knows what people go through day to day, you hear on the news people are killing themselves and I want to help people get the right help to listen to my song before doing something bad
This finished 22/01/2019
Bobby latheron

This is my third song
ONE LYRICS
Verse 1

If we all stand together we
can beat this thing as
one before the world disappear
forever and the enemy has won

If we all stand together
we can stop the bombs
stop the war where is
the love between us what
are we fighting for

Chorus

Where is the love where's the
unity is not what god
extended us to be if
we are one we can heal
this broken world we be
back where we belong if
we keep on standing strong
we can be one

Verse 2

As people die around us
I ask have we done
enough as the rich chose
to ignore them and share
they tear of blood as one

As children is left alone
with no one to hold
and no one to love
them as the world get
torn apart we need to mend
they broken hearts

Chorus

Where is the love where's the
unity is not what god extended
us to be if we
are one we can heal
this broken world we be
back where we belong if
we keep on standing strong
we can be one

Verse 3

The unity for the whole
universe leave the darkness behind
and head for the sun
we need to ask ourselves
the question

Wheres the love for this world

Chorus

Where is the love where's
the unity is not what god
extended us to be if we
are one we can heal
this broken world we be
back where we belong if
we keep on standing strong
we can be one

This song is about the Manchester bombing I think we all should come all together and love for other instead of killing people or bombing our country we need all to become one for the world.
Finished on 22/06/2019
Bobby latheron

This is my fourth one
BUBBLEGUM LYRICS

MY TIME TO FLY HAS JUST BEGUN
MY TIME TO FINALLY BE SOMEONE
AND BY THE TIME THAT IVE MADE NUMBER ONE
YOU'LL BE STUCK ON MY SHOE LIKE A BUBBLEGUM

IM GLAD IVE FINALLY FOUND THE LIGHT
FOUND THE STRENGTH INSIDA ME TO FIGHT
ITS WHO'LL SLEEP ALONE AT NIGHT
WHILE IM CHILLIN n POPPIN ON A BUBBLEGUM

i first saw the light
When you torn me apart
You thought I would run
Run straight for your heart

I ran for the hills
No I never looked back
Now I opened my eyes, I Found someone new
Im at the top of their list now
So Screw you

Cause my

MY TIME TO FLY HAS JUST BEGUN
MY TIME TO FINALLY BE SOMEONE
AND BY THE TIME THAT IVE MADE NUMBER ONE
YOU'LL BE STUCK ON MY SHOE LIKE A BUBBLEGUM

IM GLAD IVE FINALLY FOUND THE LIGHT
FOUND THE STRENGTH INSIDA ME TO FIGHT
ITS WHO'LL SLEEP ALONE AT NIGHT
WHILE IM CHILLIN n POPPIN ON A BUBBLEGUM
CHILLIN n POPPIN ON A BUBBLEGUM
CHILLIN n POPPIN ON A BUBBLEGUM

I feel like a star shining brightly in the sky
While your stuck in the shadows
Still questioning why

Your sleeping alone
With only your pillow to love
Now I've moved on. Im so glad that your gone
Now Im loving myself Im number one

MY TIME TO FLY HAS JUST BEGUN
MY TIME TO FINALLY BE SOMEONE
AND BY THE TIME THAT IVE MADE NUMBER ONE
YOU'LL BE STUCK ON MY SHOE LIKE A

BUBBLEGUM

IM GLAD IVE FINALLY FOUND THE LIGHT
FOUND THE STRENGTH INSIDA ME TO FIGHT
ITS WHO'LL SLEEP ALONE AT NIGHT
WHILE IM CHILLIN n POPPIN ON A BUBBLEGUM

MY TIME TO FLY HAS JUST BEGUN
MY TIME TO FINALLY BE SOMEONE
AND BY THE TIME THAT IVE MADE NUMBER ONE
YOU'LL BE STUCK ON MY SHOE LIKE A BUBBLEGUM

IM GLAD IVE FINALLY FOUND THE LIGHT
FOUND THE STRENGTH INSIDA ME TO FIGHT
ITS WHO'LL SLEEP ALONE AT NIGHT
WHILE IM CHILLIN n POPPIN ON A BUBBLEGUM
CHILLIN n POPPIN ON A BUBBLEGUM
CHILLIN n POPPIN ON A BUBBLEGUM
CHILLIN n POPPIN ON A BUBBLEGUM
CHILLIN n POPPIN ON A BUBBLEGUM

this song is about is about two people being together one getting hurt and then showing them they have moved on by chewing on a bubblegum and throwing that bubblegum out and that they are happy now.
This finished on the 22/04/2019
Bobby latheron

This is my fifth song

Wake Me Up

Im looking at myself
in the dressing room mirror
I wipe my make-up off
And all I see is sin

Losing my grip
as reality fades
The Ground falls away
as the voices are saying

Too young to die
too old for this
Its taking me over
Gets harder to resist

Wake me up
I need you now
Wake me up
Theres no way out
Wake me up
Ive had enough
Wake me up
I need you now

I need you now

Im stuck inside a dream
Drowning in deep waters
Just holding on
As I step back from the edge

Shattered glass surrounds me
I might hurt myself
I thought someone could save me
But I need to save myself

Wake me up
I need you now
Wake me up
There's no way out
Wake me up
Ive had enough
Wake me up
I need you now

I need you
Im drowning
I need you now
I need you
Cos Im fallin down
I need you now
I need you now

 You saved me from my demons
Freed me from my chains
An Angel came to me
And repented all my sins

I was standing on the ledge
It was you who talked me In
Now I'm back from the edge
I won't go back………… again

Wake me up
I need you now
Wake me up
There's no way out

Wake me up
Ive had enough
Wake me up
I need you now

This songs about helping yourself before you fall down and pick yourself up, getting rid of any bad thoughts.
This finished 22/07/2019
Bobby latheron

On March 11th 2019 the group and I visited central park's restaurant for a social evening. This social group was Shannon's first group session with Autism Matters. However this individual was no first time acquaintance, during my years at art collage she was also a student there.

I couldn't believe we barely socialized during our time at art as our personalities click well.

Although through college she had her friends/social group and I had mine which barely interlink.

I wish I had the opportunity to build a friendship with her back then because now we are like best friends. We go to fun fairs, concerts etc. I cant wait to see where our friendships takes us.

I am interviewing Shannon on some questions on autism.

1. What is your understanding of autism?

    My understanding of autism is that autism is a neurological disability that effects a individuals comprehension, mental/stress, social and emotional behaviors.

2. What do you think of people with autism and how does it effect peoples lives?

> I think people with autism are easily misunderstood by society, even family and friends. On the positive side I think people with autism are interesting, as I always say "Autism is like a snowflake, we all share similar behaviors however no two are identically the same".
>
> I think autism effects peoples lives in the sense that it is not as easy for them to have normalize life, such as relationships being independent. Also having a low thresh hold when it comes to stress, anxiety and coping/processing your emotions and trying to communicate/understand others. Additionally, I think it can be extremely stressful for people having to cope with people that have autism. Such as trying to understand and figuring out what they need in order to cope within life.

3. What do you think of me and my autism?

> From what I have noticed, I think that your autism effects you in these areas:
>
> Trying to communicate and voice your feelings with others.
>
> Unintentionally speaking loud and getting over excitable.
>
> Repetition, such as in convocation. Meaning it's hard for you to get to the point without having to repeat yourself.

However I like you just the way you are. Your funny, emotional and very caring person, and I also to struggle in these areas at times.

4. Do you think it's easy for people for autism to get a job?

yes and no, for the more able people with autism (high functioning) it is possible for them to find employment. However, they are always gonna need some level of understanding and support around them from their employer and coworkers around them, in order for them to maintain a job without too much stress.

This was finished on 21/07/2019

I have now been with Sports Village Gym for about 4 years for and about 1 year I have grown a friendships with all the personal gym teachers. They are all lovely and look after their members for about 3 month. I have been working with one of the staff 1 to 1 for personal gym session, I enjoy the sessions. He doesn't do something you can't do, he just says take your time and do as many as you can; we have good laughs together.

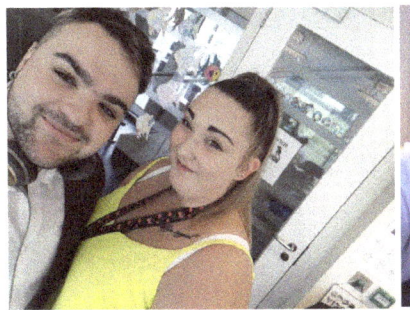

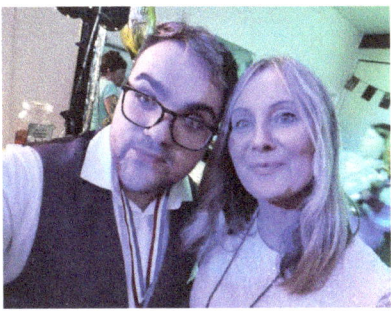

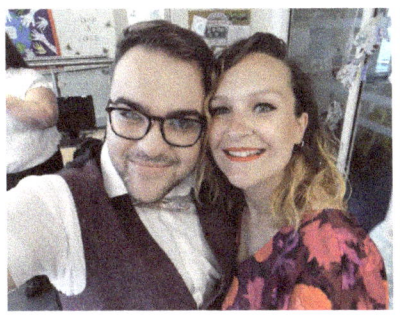

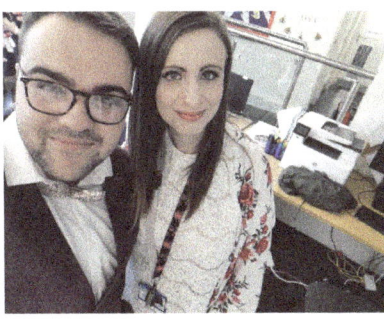

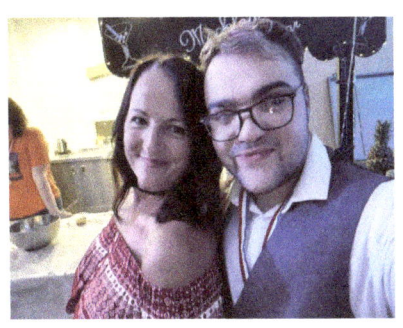

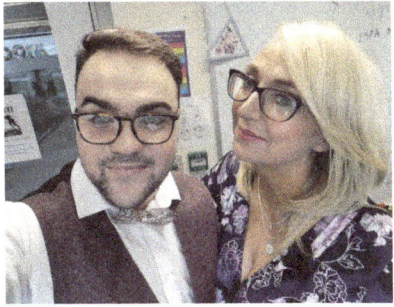

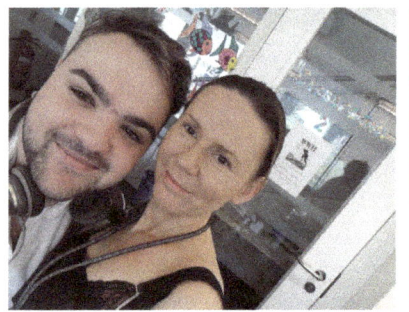

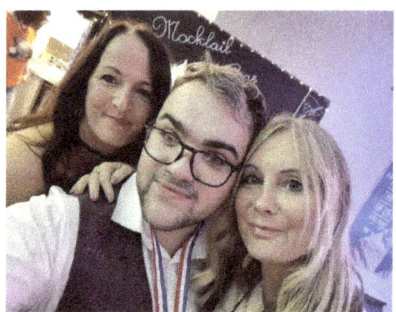

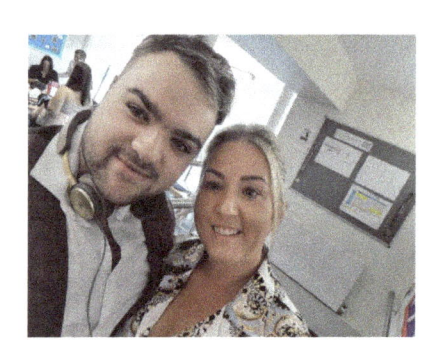

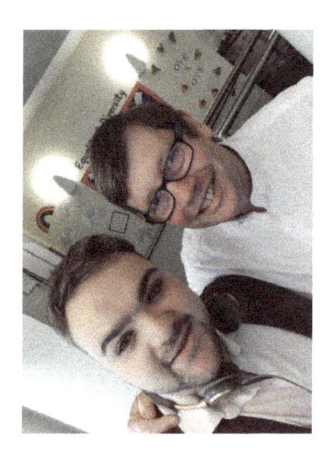

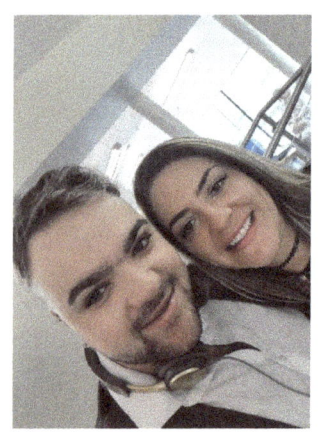

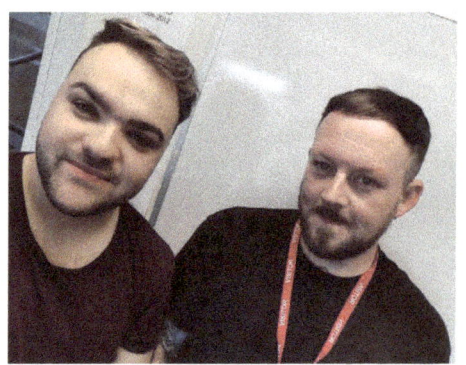

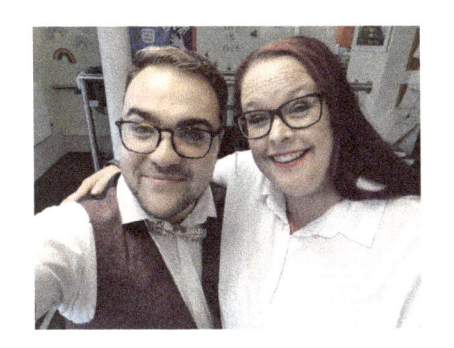

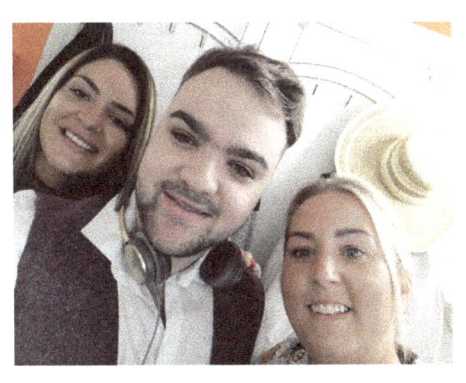

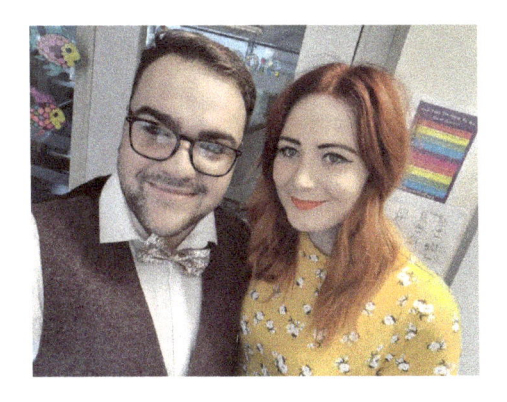

Espa 2017-2019

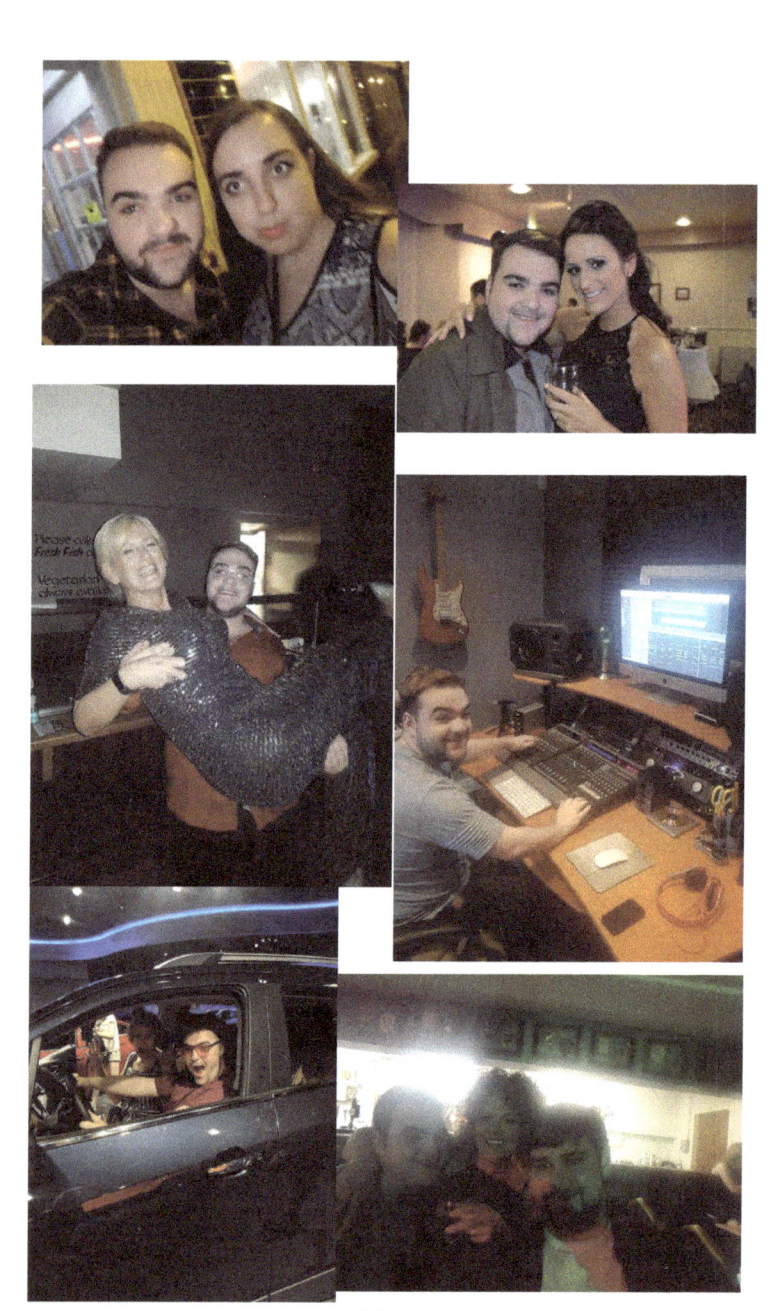

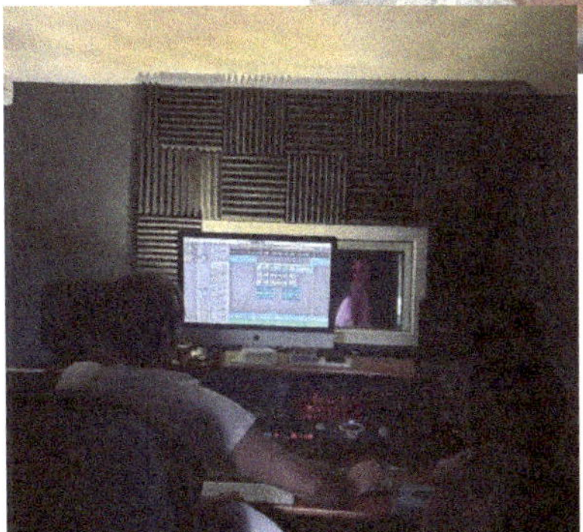

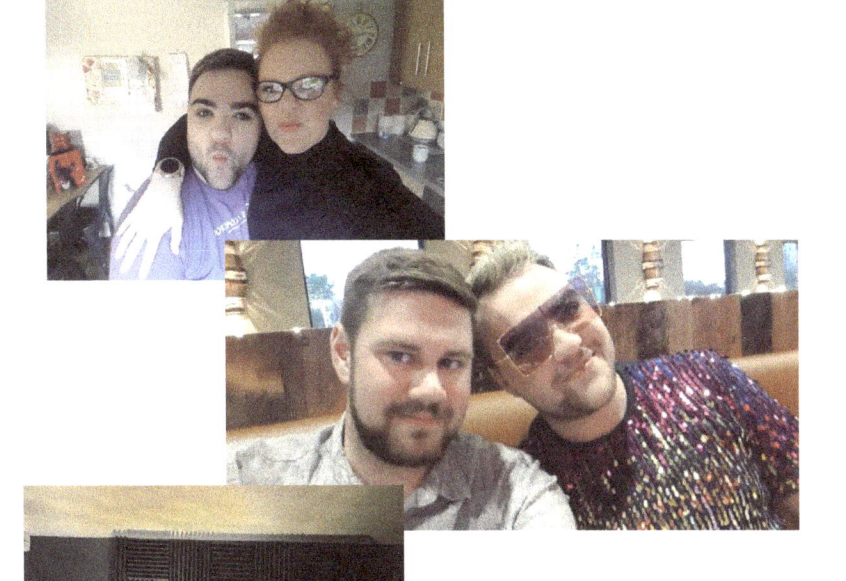

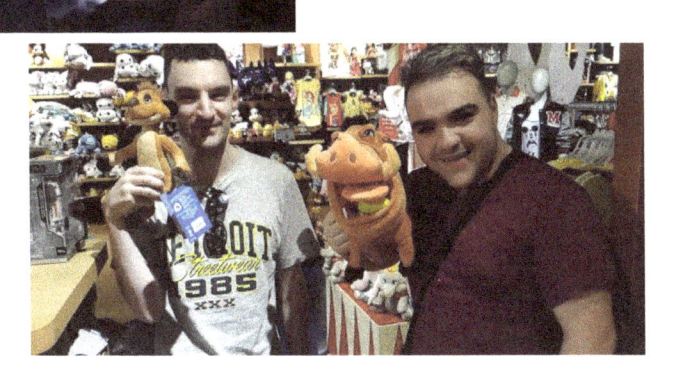

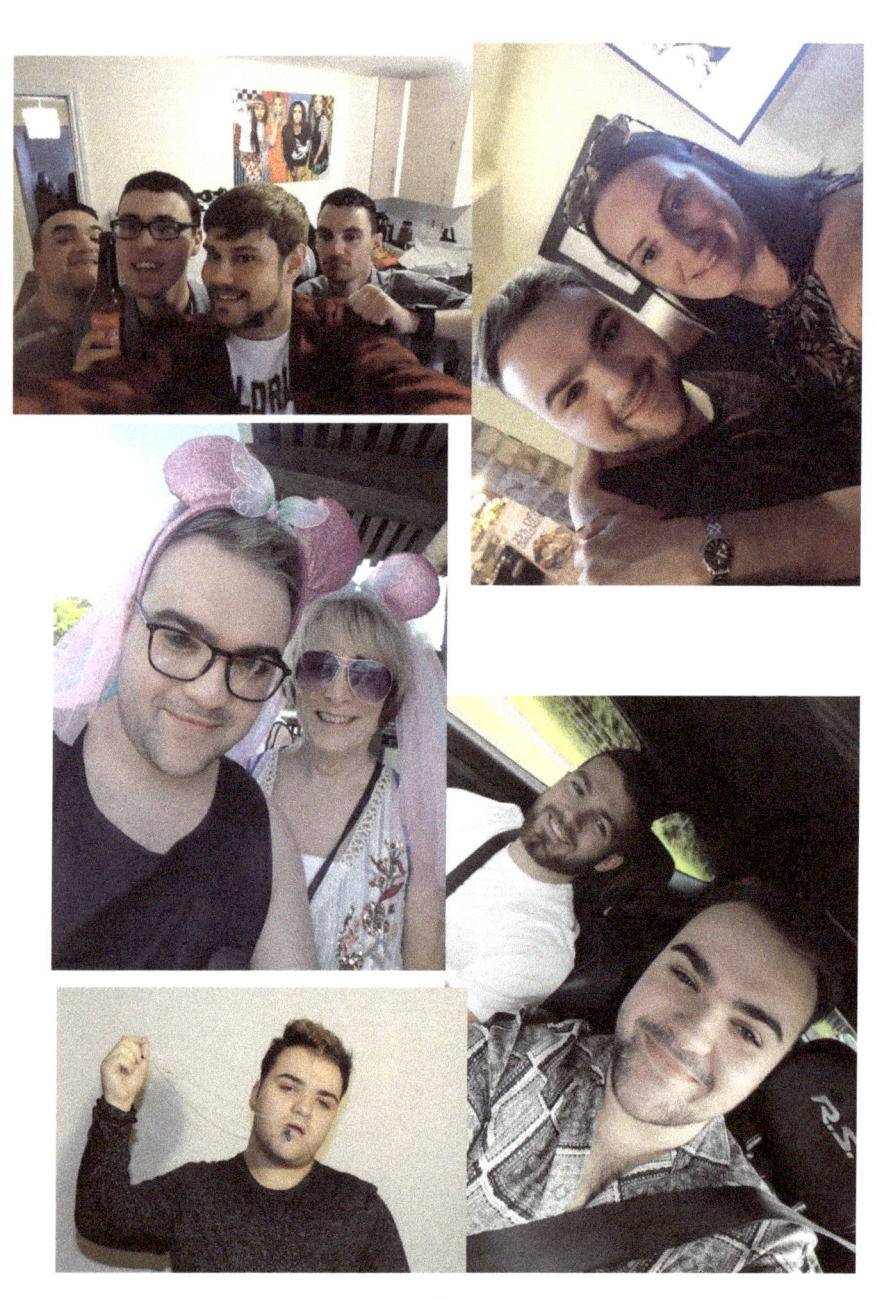

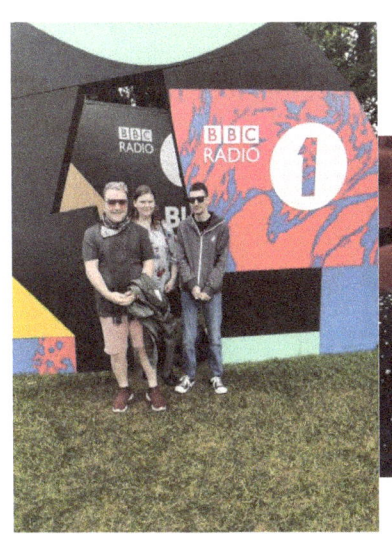

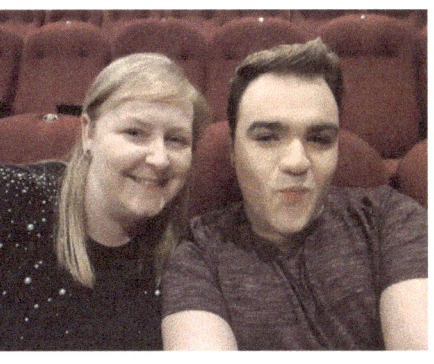

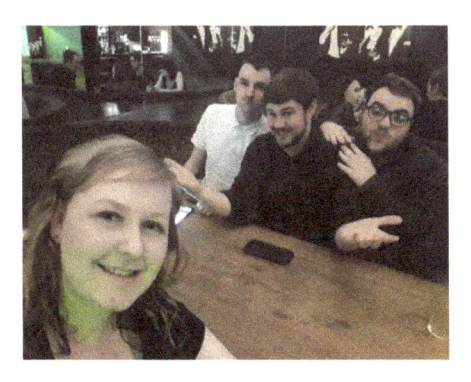

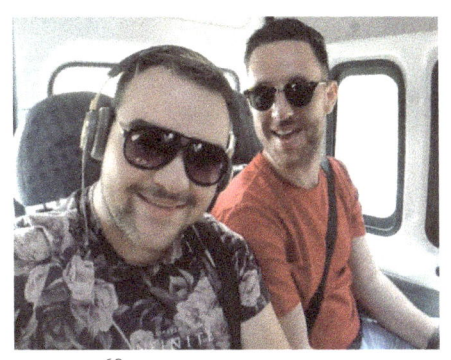

Autism
matters

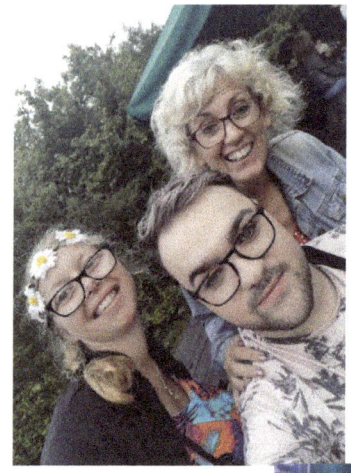

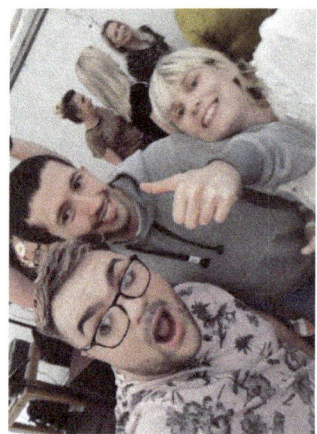

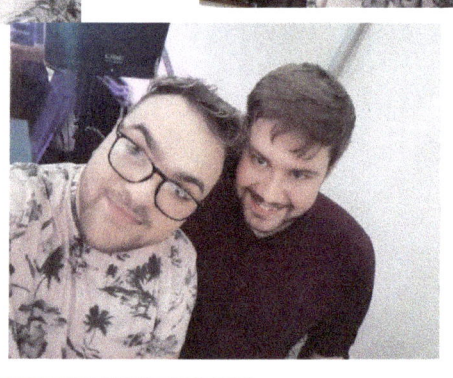

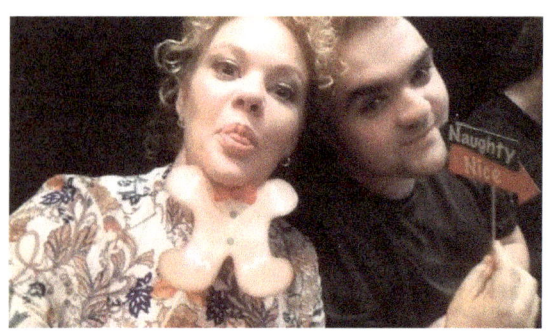

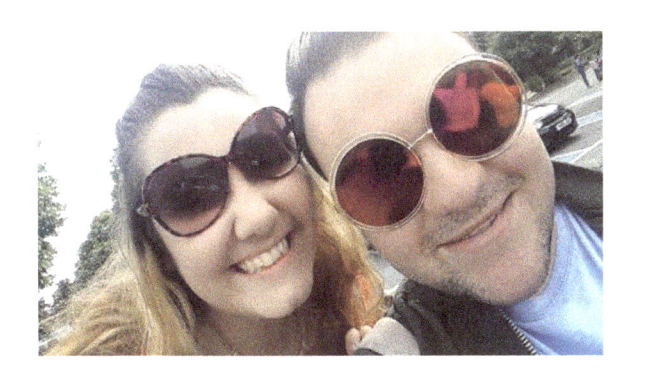

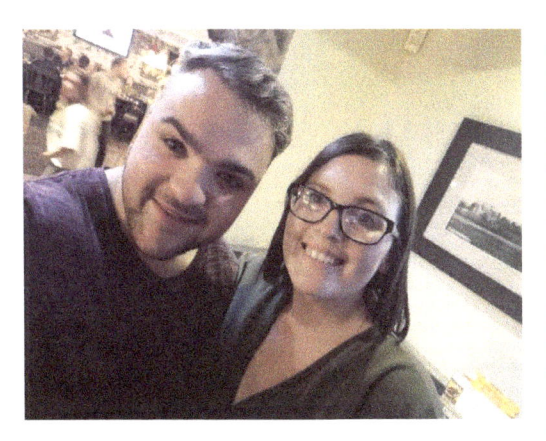

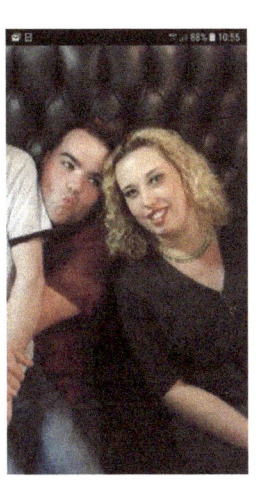

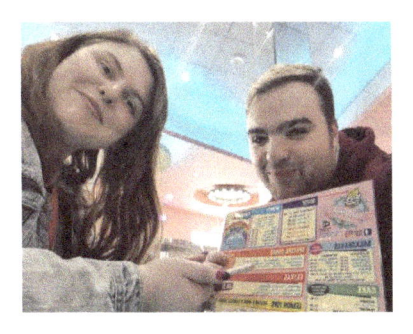

family

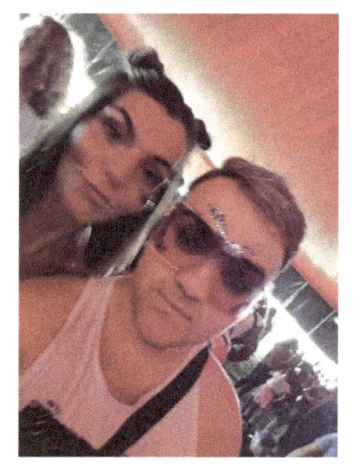

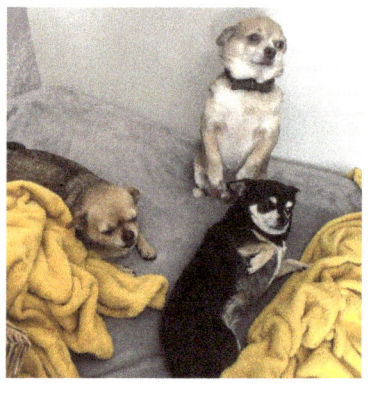

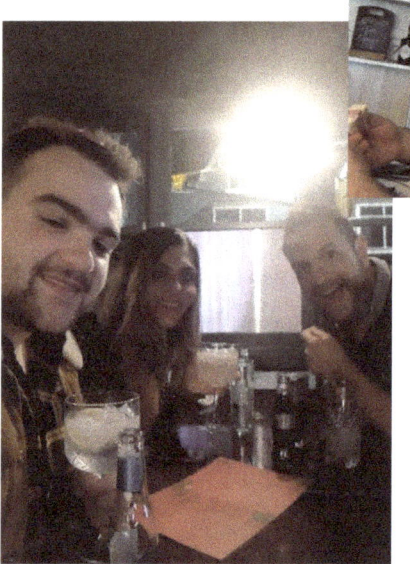

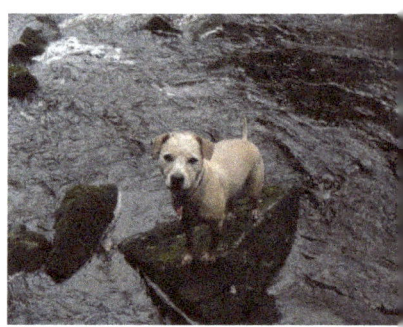

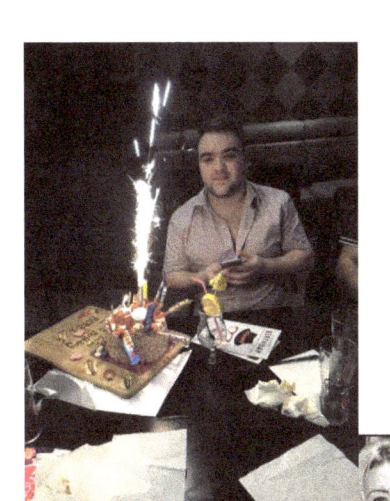

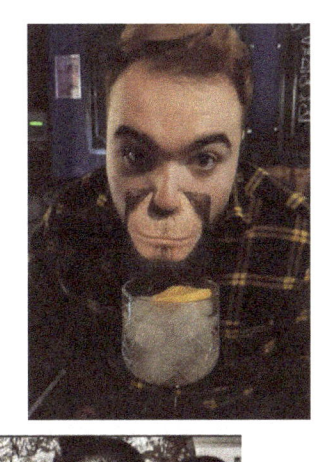

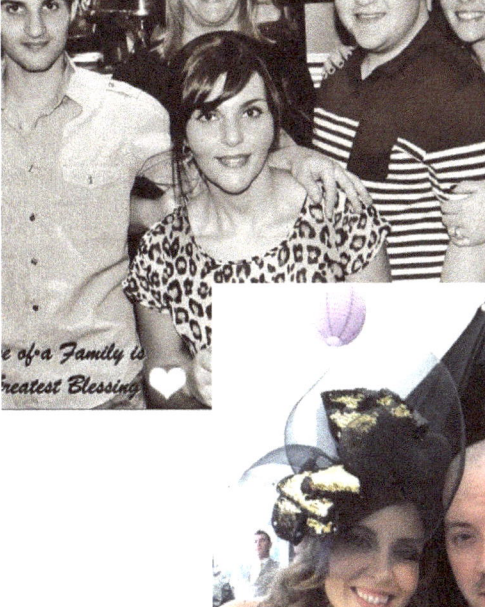

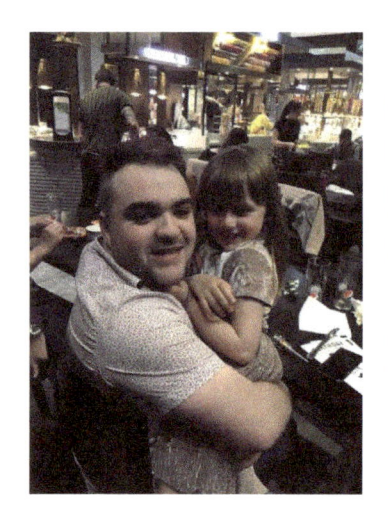

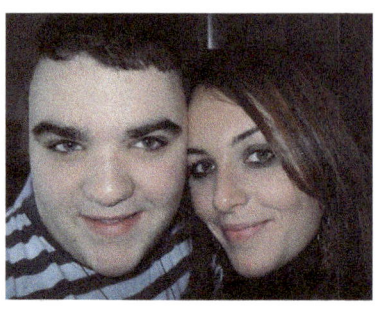

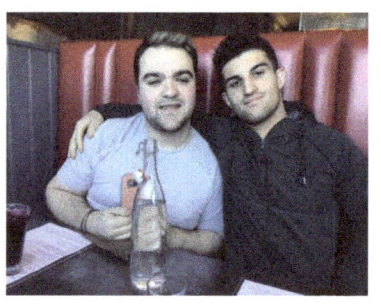

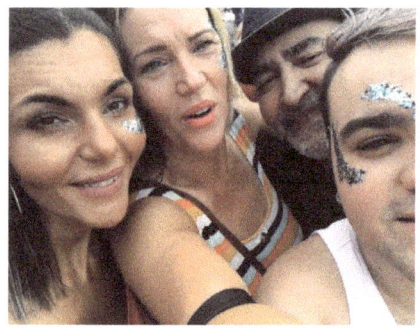

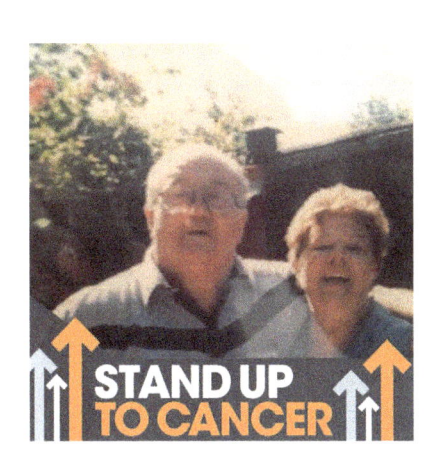

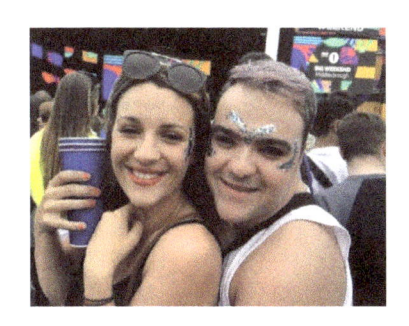

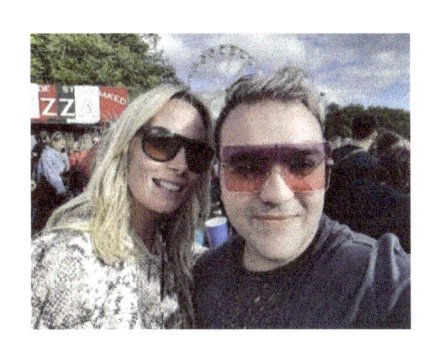

Between The Two by Bobby Latheron

CAST:

Anna – best friend of Lynne and mother of Matthew

Lynne – mother of bobby

Matthew friend of bobby

Dan M (friends of Johnny and Simon bowel)

Suzy (bff of bobby and Matthew girlfriend)

Dan – Peter Sande

Johnny – Hugh Hackman, Nicky Plarke

Leanne – barmaid

Natalie – makeup artist

Charlotte – Charlotte Brosby

Ferry, dani dye – Shannon

The registrar, lady baba – Angela

Vicky – cilla, char

Richard – rick

Counselor, Hugh mam's – Angela

PC Amy - Amy

Nurse poppy sunflower - Alex

Judge Chris franks - Howard

Hugh's wife - Kate

Hugh's sisters - jess, Jessie

Bobby, Anna, Matthew and Lynne all lived together in one house Anna was divorce mam and Lynne was to Anna was married to David Peckham and Lynne was married to Phillip Scarfield

SCENE 1

(It was the day of bobby's birthday and his mam Lynne got bobby a watch with his name on it)

Lynne: "bobby wakkkke upppp"

Bobby: "yes mam what do you want"

Lynne: I made you some birthday breakfast come and open your presents before we go to America"

Bobby: okkkk mam coming hold on"

(Bobby went down stairs to see his mam made him some breakfast)

Lynne: "happy birthday son love ya"

Bobby: "thanks mam love ya too"

(Bobby opened his present his mam got him and she wrapped them all up with rose gold glitter wrapping up paper)

Bobby: "I love them all thanks mam"

Lynne: "it's ok son there you go"

(There was a knock on the door and it was Matthew and Anna)

Anna and Matthew: "HAPPY BIRTHDAYYYY YOU LITTLE DIVA"

Bobby: "thanks bitches love ya lots"

(Anna and Matthew given bobby a card for his birthday)

Bobby: "thank you, you didn't have to"

(There was written on the card and it said)

To bobby happy birthday and see you when you come back from America for your first singing lesson it was no one but peter Sande.

2 weeks later when they came back.

(It was the day of bobby's first singing lessons with peter Sande)

Bobby: "MAAAAAAAAAAM"

(Bobby's mam ran as fast as she can to his room and she said)

Lynne: " you ok son?"

Bobby: "yes mam but today the day I meet my idol aaaaaahhhhh"

Lynne: "son you scared me I thought I lost my hair"

Bobby: " "mam your looks like normal as always"

Lynne: "thanks son for the comment"

(Anna and Matthew came for a cup of tea)

(Anna and Lynne where having a glass of gin like they always do)

Anna: (said to Lynne) I wish I was married to Johnny jeep)

Lynne: (laughed at the top of her lungs) "hahahaha you wish keep on dreaming"

Anna: "thanks lynne for that"

Lynne: "sorry but you know its true lol"

Anna: "you're right lol"

(Matthew and bobby were talking about stuff)

Matthew: "you looking forward to your singing lesson"

Bobby: "hell yeah can't wait to meet peter but very nervous to sing to him"

Matthew: "you be fine just be yourself here drink this gin before you go and you be fine"

Bobby: "ok mate thanks I don't know what I wouldn't do without a friend like you can you do me a favour"

Matthew: "what do you want bobby lol"

Bobby: "will you take me for my singing lesson please can't drive while I had a drink please"

Matthew: "of cause mate anything for you"

Bobby: "cheers mate"

Lynne: "look bobby you know you past you driving lessons?"

Bobby: "yes mam why what's up?"

Lynne: "well here you go?"

(Lynne given bobby some car keys)

(We all looked at the window and there was a car for me it was a fiat 500 in bubble gum purple just want he wanted)

(Bobby starts to cry)

Bobby:" "mam thanks you're the best I love ya xxx"

Lynne: "you welcome love ya to x"

(Matthew took bobby in his mini soft top)

Bobby: "you ready to take me mate"

Matthew: "yeah mate just get my keys hold on"

Bobby: "ok mate"

Bobby and Matthew: "bye mam love ya's

Lynne and Anna: bye love ya's"

(Matthew and bobby were cruising in the car with the roof down singing top of their lungs to Nastacia left outside blone also dancing to the song)

SCENE 2

(Bobby gets out of Matthew car)

Bobby: "mate will you pick me up at 3 please?"

Matthew: "ok mate I'll give you a text when am 10 minutes away"

Bobby: "cheers matey see ya then"

(Bobby knocks on the door and peter opens it)

Bobby: "ahhhhhhhhh"

(Bobby falls into peter's arms)

Peter: "are you ok bobby there"

Bobby: "yeah just tell me am your mysteries boy to me"

Peter: "oh oh oh bobby you are my mysteries boy but your body next to mine"

Bobby: "ok am ok now am ready to start"

(Peter and bobby are talking about what bobby what's peter to help him with)

Peter: "so bobby what are you here to see me about?"

Bobby: "well peter I like to sing but I rather be more of a song writer because as you know I have autism but I keep all my emotion to myself but I like to write them in my songs"

Peter: "ok so what would you like me to do?"

Bobby: "I want you to sing them for me if that's all right with you"

Peter: "yeah ok then let's get started what song you would like to do first"

Bobby: "well peter I have already finish some lyrics and the name of the song is called happy ending would you like to read it"

Peter: "yes please if you don't mind"

(Bobby gives Peter the lyrics to look at)

Peter: "OMG these lyrics are shamzing!"

Bobby: "aww thanks peter that means a lot to me"

(Bobby's two hours came up and there was someone waiting to see peter next)

Peter: "so bobby our time is up how you want to book your sessions then"

Bobby: "can we do one a fortnight on a Thursday at 1 to 3"

Peter: "yeah see you then"

Bobby: "ok peter well bye see ya later"

(Knock knock)

Peter: "hello Suzy how you doing"

(Bobby turned around and he was happy to see the girl who came in)

Bobby: "aaaaaahhhhh Suzy it's been to long how are you doing?"

Suzy: "am great how are you doing bobby"

Bobby: "great it's been to long we need a catch up"

Suzy: "yeah I know what you doing tomorrow"

Bobby: "nothing why you want to catch up like"

Suzy: "yeah go on then why not"

(Bobby and Suzy were like sisters in secondary but lost touch when they went to college)

(The next day bobby and Suzy met at the peppermill cafe for some lunch)

Bobby: "so Suzy what are you doing now with yourself"

Suzy: "I am working in a library"

Bobby: "great I bet you love it"

Suzy: "yeah it's great job"

Bobby: "so are you seeing anyone at the minute then"

Suzy: "no I am single bit I am looking why"

(Bobby showed a picture of Matthew to Suzy)

Bobby: "what do you think of my friend Matthew?"

Suzy: "he looks cute he looks a bit like Justin Piber just my type but I bet he has a girlfriend though"

Bobby: "no he is single"

Suzy: oh right"

(Bobby went home and spoke to Matthew about Suzy)

Bobby: "MATTHEW"

Matthew: "what's wrong bobby"

Bobby: "nowt come here got something to ask you"

Matthew: "ok coming now"

Bobby: "Mathew my good friend who I haven't seen in years in single and I would like for you to meet her"

Matthew: "ok then set it up then"

Bobby: I will I got to go now for my 4th singing lessons"

(Bobby arrived at peter house for his lesson)

Bobby: "hi peters how are you"

Peter: "I'm great thanks"

(Peter was in the studio singing bobby's song through the rose gold glitter microphone)

(Before bobby went home he had something to ask peter)

Bobby: "peter can I ask you something"

Peter: "yeah go on then what do you want to ask me"

Bobby: "are you single"

Peter: "yes why do you ask?"

Bobby: "are you gay or straight"

Peter: "I am gay why you do ask"

Bobby: "can I ask you for a date"

Peter: "yeah I was going to ask you but I was scared too"

Bobby: "aww you so cute like a pie"

(So bobby and peter and Matthew and Suzy went on their first double date)

(Peter got bobby some multi-colour glitter roses)

Bobby: "aww thanks peter there are gorgeous you didn't have to"

Peter: "you welcome and you are my date so I want to get you them"

(Before Suzy came for her date bobby and Matthew went to the flower shop to get Suzy some Matthew got her some pink roses)

(Suzy came and Matthew gives her the flowers)

Suzy: "thank you, you didn't have to they are gorgeous"

Matthew: "no I want to and you are welcome"

(Bobby had the chicken salad, peter had the chicken Parmo, Matthew had a burger and Suzy had the fish and chips)

(Peter and Matthew went to the bar to get the drinks in)

Bobby: "omg peter how did you know I like gin well I looked on your Facebook and found you liked it so I got you it"

Bobby: "thanks"

(Matthew got Suzy lemonade and vodka)

Suzy: "thanks Matt"

Matthew: "you welcome"

SCENE 3

(7 months down the line peter had to ask bobby something)

(Peter is crying to bobby)

Peter: "bobby I have to go and live in Florida"

Bobby: "what you breaking up with me like"

Peter: "I want you to come and live with me, because I love you so much"

(Bobby ran out of his lesson to his house)

Bobby: "maaaaaaammmm he is moving to Florida and he asks me to move with me, but I don't know what to do I don't want to live you behind"

(Lynne slaps bobby)

Bobby: "ouch mam what was that for"

Lynne: "what the hell you got a nice man there who told you he loved you and he wants to show you the world and you walked out"

Bobby: "yeah because it means me leaving you behind"

Lynne: "look son I love you but I don't want to hold you back I come for visits lol"

(Bobby told Anna, Matthew and Suzy about the news)

Bobby: "guys I got something to tell you"

Anna and Matthew: (at the same time as always) "what wrong?"

Bobby: "guys can you stop doing that at the same time"

Suzy: "what's up matey?"

Bobby: "well peter ask me to move in with him"

Matthew Suzy and Anna: "OMG AHHH WHEN"

Bobby: "this Saturday but to Florida

Anna: "oh well I think it's a great idea"

Suzy: "I think it is a great idea but we will miss you"

Matthew: "well I don't think it's a good idea he is taking my friend and my brother away"

(Matthew was so upset he ran off)

(They were all looking for Matthew but bobby found him in the tree house they used to go in as in kids)

(Bobby was trying to talk to Matthew in the tree house)

Bobby: "Matthew please can we talk about this please

Matthew: "no"

Bobby: "well am going to speak and I hope you listen, he loves me and I love him too, I never forget you, you are my brother from other mother and my best friend, it is hard for me too you know saying goodbye to you"

(Matthew came round)

(Matthew and bobby hugged it out)

Matthew: "I am really going to miss you, you know"

Bobby: "I miss you too, but we can always Skype and talk I'm only a call away even though I am thousand miles away"

Matthew: "true lol"

(Bobby ring up peter to say)

Bobby: "peter lets go and do it on our next chapter of our lives"

Peter: "ok let's do it I love you"

Bobby: "I love you to"

SCENE 4

(2 year later bobby and peter came back home for a week holiday we went to the cinemas with Matthew and Suzy and we watched a classic dirty lancing)

(Peter was acting funny, he asked Matthew for a private word)

Peter: "Matthew can I show you something"

Matthew: "yeah mate what do you want to show me"

(Peter pulls out a ring)

Peter: "do you like the ring am going to ask bobby to marry me I've done a little clip before the film has started do you like it"

Matthew: "yeah mate I think he is going to like it"

(Bobby, Suzy and Matthew went to the screen for the film)

Bobby: "Matthew where has peter gone to"

Matthew: "he just went to get something out of the car"

Bobby: "ok Matt"

(When bobby went in the screen all his friends and family were there he looked shocked but happy to see them all)

(5 minutes before the film started bobby was shocked to see peter on the screen, with the song rude playing in the clip by magic)

(the clip was quite funny, peter asked bobby mam's friend Anna if he can ask her a question and she shut the door on his face, but lynne opened the door and she he asked her the question and she nodded her head yes about something)

(the clip ended and peter was there with thousand for roses multicolour roses, bobby was crying, peter asked bobby a question and he bend down and pulled this gorgeous rose gold)

(Peter said to bobby)

Peter: "bobby will you marry me please"

Bobby: "………………………………."

SCENE 5

Peter: "well bobby what is your answer"

Bobby: "yeah of course I marry you with all my heart"

(Lynne give bobby I kiss and hugged peter)

Lynne: "I love you both so much"

Anna Matthew Suzy: "congrats guys"

(Bobby was in happy tears thanks guys so much)

(Bobby and peter kiss)

SCENE 6

(Bobby was thinking of a Facebook page for his music)

Bobby: "what shall I call my Facebook page mmmmmmm?"

(5 minutes later bobby thought of the idea for his page)

Bobby: "I will call my page diva records north east

6 months later

(while bobby and Suzy was planning the wedding and the hen party bobby got a called of Simon bowel)

Bobby: "hello who is speaking please?"

Simon: "well hello bobby my name is Simon Bowell"

(Bobby looked shocked and Suzy said)

Suzy: "what is wrong bobby?"

Bobby: "Mr Simon bowel is on the phone"

Suzy: "ahhhhhh what does he want like"

Bobby: "I don't know am speaking to you duh"

Suzy: "oh yeah well ask him then"

Bobby: "am going to lol"

(Bobby was back on the phone to Simon bowel)

Bobby: "yes Simon what do you want from me"

Simon: "so bobby I have seen your page on Facebook and I have to say is can I sign you up to my company"

Bobby: "ahhhhhhhh"

(Bobby falls on the floor and Suzy says)

Suzy: "Bobby are you ok"

Bobby: "I'm fine it just Simon asked me to be part of his team"

Suzy: "ahhhhhhh great what you going to say"

Bobby: "Simon sign me up baby cakes"

(Bobby went back to his mam's with Suzy and there was a surprise)

Lynne Anna Matthew peter: "congrats"

(Suzy told them about the good news)

(We celebrated by playing games music drinks and pizza)

(Bobby said to peter with his arms around him)

Bobby: "I'm so glad to have you in my life and my friend and family it has been a great week but we better be getting packed for to go back home tomorrow"

Peter: "you're right darling let's go and pack"

(The day after bobby give his mam and Anna a kiss goodbye before he had to go to the airport)

(Matthew and Suzy took bobby and peter to the airport)

Bobby and peter: "bye guys see you soon"

Matthew and Suzy: "bye guys safe journey"

(But peter and bobby had a little surprise for Matthew and Suzy on they 3rd anniversary)

Peter: "bobby tell them the good news"

Matthew: "what is it bobby"

Bobby: "you're coming with us we packed your bags xx"

Matthew and Suzy: "ahhhh you guys thanks"

SCENE 7

(3 days later setting in our house)

(Bobby and Suzy where thinking where to go for the hen party)

Bobby: "Suzy let's go here girlfriend"

Suzy: "let's go bff"

(Bobby called all of mine and Suzy friends bitches we going for my hen party to the love party villa in Mallorca)

(Bobby and Suzy went back to England while peter had in stag do with Matthew and their friends)

Bobby: mam and Anna have you packed yet"

Lynne and Anna: "nearly just getting our make-up and our wrinkle cream"

(Bobby and Suzy laughed)

(Bobby and Suzy called all our friends to say if there are at the airport yet)

(Bobby called his other bff and make-up artist Natalie and said)

Bobby: "Natalie you all girls there yet"

Natalie: "yeah we are here just waiting for the party to come"

Bobby: "we on our way just 5 minutes away"

(We all got there safe and we had an hour to kill so we went to McDonald for our dinner)

(We all got on the plane ok bobby was sat with his bff's Natalie and Suzy)

(We all had 5 hours to go to land)

(Lynne and Anna were drunk as hell they got everyone drinks on the plane and they both got up and danced to Whitney Nouton one of her song"

(The security guards had to come and tell them to be quiet Lynne and Anna we're trying to kiss them so they told them to get out of first class and they put them in normal seats)

Cilla: "hello ladies can you both be quiet please"

Lynne: - "how about you get us the drinks love we having a party here"

Cilla: - "look lady all I ask was to keep it down please that's all ok"

Anna: - "look love just go away because we are first class ok"

(Bobby and the girls looks and laughs at them getting told off)

Cilla: "well ladies for since you talking to me like that you are getting moved"

(Anna and Lynne had to be moved)

(Bobby and the rest of the girls laughed they heads off)

(But then bobby and Suzy and Natalie got up and danced to Ceyonce songs everyone was cheering us on)

(Anna and Lynne said to the guards)

Anna and Lynne: "well hello there you sexy guards, beautiful they making noises now"

(And they really good at it and they not even sorry lol)

(We got to the airport and everyone got their suitcases but bobby we had to wait an hour and a half)

Natalie: "what's wrong bobby"

Bobby: (crying) "my suitcase is missing and the bus has left us"

(Then bobby got a phone call of peter saying I got you and all your friends a surprise)

Peter: "look outside bobby"

(Bobby and the gang looked outside and there was a rose gold glitter party bus with gin and dance poles inside of the bus)

(Bobby said to peter)

Bobby: "we can't go because my suitcase isn't here"

Peter: "hahahaha I told the security to hold it back until I rang you up with the surprise lol got you"

Bobby: "I will get you back love you"

Peter and Matthew: "yeah whatever lol"

(We got to the villa after an hour of travelling)

(It was 11 at night so Lynne and Anna went to bed)

(Bobby and all the girls were just having drinks and talking)

(And bobby said to all the girls)

Bobby: "Natalie and Suzy come here quick I got a plan you want to be in the game"

Natalie and Suzy: "yeah what game is it"

Bobby: "get all the girls together me you Suzy and Natalie get some chocolate and cream mix it in we go in the room where Anna and lynne are sleeping in tell them to wake up and splash the cream and chocolate on their face after what they did on the plane"

Natalie and Suzy: "yeah let's do it"

Bobby: "Natalie also gets the girls to get on the balcony we lead them outside and they will drop water bombs on them and they land in the pool it will be class"

(The plan was working great and they did end in the pool)

All the girls: "hahahaha that what you get after embracing us on the plane"

Bobby: "this is going to be the craziest 4 days of my life

SCENE 8

(2nd day of the lads stag do)

(Bobby ranged up Matthew and said to him)

Bobby: "Matthew will you do me a big favour please"

Matthew: "what is it like?"

Bobby: "so after what peter did to me in the airport, I want you to get him a jump of the plane and get all of his mates to take a video off him screaming, because doesn't like height"

Matthew: "Matthew I'll get on it now"

(Matthew told all the guy's about the idea and they were all laughing and said mint can't wait lol)

(Matthew rang up the place to see if they can do it today, and the person said yes bring him down)

(Matthew told everyone and said they were going out for drinks but really they were getting ready to take peter for the ride of his life)

(Matthew told peter)

Matthew: "peter I have to fold blind your eyes because bobby got you a surprise is that ok"

Peter: "yeah ok then"

(Matthew then blind fold his eyes and they went to the grass were they plane was waiting for peter)

(Peter then went up with the plane and the guy hooked him onto him and said to Peter will you take your blind fold of please)

(Peter said ok and he saw how high he was and the guy said "here we go")

Peter: "no wait please AHHHHHHHH HEEEELPP MMMMEEEE"

All the lads: "HAHAHAHA"

(Peter got on the ground and he had a phone call of bobby)

Peter: "you won't believe what I did babe"

Bobby: "what did you jump out of a plane?"

Peter: "yes, but how did you know"

Bobby: "well babe I was the one who planned it after what you did to me in the airport, ha-ha I told ya I get you back"

Peter: "well you did babe, I can't wait to marry you"

Bobby: "I can't wait to marry you"

SCENE 9

(It was the 3rd day of the girl's hen's party)

(Peter called Suzy and Natalie by face time and said to them)

Peter: "take bobby to flares for his last day before the wedding in couple weeks"

Natalie and Suzy: "ok we will make it good for him"

(Natalie and Suzy got all the girls together told them the plans for tonight)

All girls: "whaooooo party"

(Natalie did all the girls make up, but did bobby's last)

Bobby: "can I have everything nude please in lipstick, lip liner, eye shadow"

Natalie: "no more nude's please, let me do your make-up"

Bobby: "ok you do what you do best"

(Natalie was finished with the make-up)

Natalie: "bobby you can open your eyes now"

(Bobby looked shocked)

Bobby: "Natalie"

Natalie: "what"

Bobby: "I look shamzing and beautiful thank you"

(Everyone got to flares and bobby was shocked where he was)

(We all were dancing and we didn't know who was the dj was but we all loved her)

Charlotte: "welcome to bobby's hen parrrttyyyy"

(She played peter Sande song mysteries girl)

(She come and join the party we all loved her)

Charlotte: "who is the lucky person then?"

Bobby: "I am xx"

(Bobby asked Charlotte a question)

Bobby: "Charlotte"

Charlotte: "yes"

Bobby: "would you like to join us for the next 2 days"

Charlotte: "yes let's get the party started can I ask my friend to come Leanne she works on the bar"

Bobby: "yeah of she can she looks lovely"

(Bobby walks up to Leanne and says)

Bobby: "hi are you Leanne Charlotte friends"

Leanne: "well yes I am and who are you"

Bobby: "my name is bobby I'm getting married to Peter Sande"

Leanne: "really aaaaaahhhhhh"

Bobby: "yeah"

Leanne: "congrats"

Bobby: "would you like to join me and my girls and now Charlotte for my hen do for the last 2 days in the villa"

Leanne: "yeah thanks for the invite

(Day 3 for the men's stag do)

(Peter talk to bobby about his school friend Dan Mortimer so bobby rings Dan and says)

Bobby: "hi Dan M my name is bobby and I'm getting married to one of your friends peter from school he said he lost touch with you when you started to work for McDonald.

Dan M: "oh yes peter he was my best mate what can I do for you.

Bobby: "his on his last day on his stag do and I would like it, if you go and surprise him, he would be so glad to see you again.

Dan M: "yes I would love to go and meet him"

Bobby: Great thank you he will love to see you again

(Bobby rings up Matthew to meet Dan at the airport)

Bobby: "Matthew peter friends coming to meet up with you for the last day, but I want it to be a surprise for him"

Matthew: "ok bobby what do you want me to do"

Bobby: "I want you to tell the lads go for a drink, and take peter with them, you go and pick Dan M up and, I want you to tell the lads that when they near the house beep so you know to hide Dan M in the closet"

Matthew: "ok bobs I'll get on it"

(Matthew told all the lads and they were on board with it)

Matthew: "oi oi peter come here lad"

Peter: "what do you want Matthew now god go and listen to baby by Justin Pieber.

Matthew: "OI OI chill out lad, all I was going to say is that the lads are going to take you to Liger Liger for some drinks on your last day".

Peter: "ok great thanks"

(The lads went and left Matthew behind)

Peter: "Matthew why aren't you coming to liger liger".

Matthew: "because I've got a hangover from last night I'll clean the house up"

Peter: "ok mate see ya later then"

Matthew: "you will"

SCENE 10

(Matthew went to pick up Dan M from the airport)

(Matthew went inside the airport with a sign saying hi welcome Dan M)

(Dan M went up to Matthew and said)

Dan M: "hi that is me, am guessing you are Matthew"

Matthew: "well I am and hello, nice to meet you"

Dan M: "you too mate, will you carry my suitcase for me please"

Matthew: "yes matey, pass it here then"

(Matthew got the suitcase from Dan M)

Matthew: wow, how heavy is this suitcase"

Dan M: "it's not that heavy, stop being a girl lol"

Matthew: "hahahahaha whatever"

(Matthew and Dan got in the car, and Matthew put on his rock music)

Dan M: "will you turn that crap music off please"

(Matthew wasn't happy)

Matthew: "well Dan what music do you like"

Dan M: "I like little bix and I want it on now"

(So Matthew but little mix on to make Dan M happy)

(Dan m is singing)

Dan M: "this is a shout out to my ex"

Matthew: "I like your singing, not"

Dan M: "at least you can listen to the song, not like screaming crap"

(Matthew and Dan M didn't really get on)

(They got back to the villa and Matthew was cleaning while Dan M was messing around while he was singing into the cleaning broom)

Matthew: "mate I have to hide you in the closet"

Dan M: "no you are not, and I do not care what bobby said to you"

(Matthew and Dan M where fighting, then Matthew taped him and hide him in the closet)

(The gang car pulled up)

Peter: "how you feeling Matthew"

Matthew: "great now thanks mate"

(Peter could hear banging from upstairs)

Peter: "Matthew what is that banging"

Matthew: "nothing mate why"

(Peter went upstairs in the closet)

Peter: "DAN M, what you doing here"

Dan M: "came to surprise you on your stag do"

Peter: "did bobby call you"

Dan M: "no he didn't why"

(Matthew stared at him)

(It was late at night and the lads and the lasses got bobby and peter a surprise)

All the Girls: "bobby come here we got a game for you"

All the Boys: "peter come here"

All the Girls and Boys: "Bobby and peter we are playing Mr and Mr"

Peter And Bobby: "hahahaha ok let's play"

(The girls recorded a video of peter and the boys recorded bobby we match all the question)

(The lads were playing a game and Dan M said)

Dan M: "peter can you remember when you met up with your ex and you kissed him"

Matthew: "what did you say Dan"

Dan M: "nothing hahahahaha"

Matthew: "peter how can you do this to bobby, you got him to come out here ask him to marry you then you kissing your ex, am telling bobby"

Peter: "Matthew please it was a mistake he came on to me, please don't tell bobby it will crush him"

(Matthew had everything recorded)

Matthew: "fine I won't tell him, but you have to tell him when we get back and tell him it was a mistake"

Peter: "fine ok I will"

Matthew: "good"

SCENE 11

(Everyone went back home, and Charlotte and Leanne went back to bobby's and peter's for the 2 weeks for the wedding)

(Bobby took his friends and family back to the airport and waved them goodbye and he said)

Bobby: "I'll see ya all in a week time for the wedding bye guys"

Everyone: "bye we love ya lot's bobby"

(Bobby went back to his house)

Bobby: "hi girls how you doing, have you seen peter anywhere"

Leanne: "yeah I think he is upstairs"

Charlotte: "yeah I think he is speaking to someone"

Bobby: "ok, so Charlotte what do you do as a job then"

Charlotte: "I am a teacher in a primary school"

Bobby: "wow, what a nice job which area do you work in"

Charlotte: "I work in London it is a really lovely school full of celebrities kids, my 2 step children goes there I am married to Chad Croeger ".

Bobby: "OMG no really or are you messing me around".

Charlotte: "no shall I show you my wedding pictures"

Bobby: "yeah please if you don't mind"

(Charlotte showed bobby the picture)

Bobby: "OMG I'm so jealous, how did you meet him then"

Charlotte: "well I got another friend called bobby from Middlesbrough and he got me and him 2 tickets to the BBC 1 radio what was 6 years ago in Middlesbrough park, and he was playing and he was singing my favourite song how you remind myself, I was that drunk I started singing and he caught my eye and said will you like to sing with me and we have been together ever since".

Bobby: "sounds like a dream come true"

Charlotte: "it was yeah"

Bobby: so Leanne what do you do as a job then"

Leanne: "well I work on the bar one's a week, cos I am also PA and also I work for a group called autism matters"

Bobby: "really I would love to work for people with autism if I weren't so busy, so Leanne are you married to anyone"

Leanne: "yeah I am also married to Bradley Looper"

Bobby: "wow, I heard he is really good looking"

Leanne: "yeah he is and also so sweet"

Bobby: "how did you meet him then?"

Leanne: "well have you heard of lady Baba"

(Bobby started to scream)

Bobby: aaaaaahhhhh, I love her she is my idol, she is why I wanted to do what I love, my songwriter"

Leanne: "well she is my best friend"

Bobby: "so how did lady Baba get you and Bradley together then?"

Leanne: "have you heard of the film called a star is a moon, and please don't scream lol"

Bobby: "yeah I love that film"

Leanne: "well she asked me to come behind the scene so I can meet them all, and then me and Bradley said hello to each other, and he asked lady Baba if that Leanne lass was single and lady Baba said yeah, and that what happened we been together for about 2 years.

Bobby: "sounds a lovely story, Leanne and Charlotte can I ask you both something"

Charlotte and Leanne: "yeah what is it bobby"

Bobby: "can they both come to my wedding and sing and Leanne will you ask lady baba to come, I just love her, ba ba ah-ah-ah! Ro mah ro-mah-mah baba oh-la-la!

(Bobby also got a question to ask Charlotte)

103

Bobby: "Charlotte will you ask chad to play too far away for me when I come down the aisle because I love that song so much and I want peter to know how much he means to me"

(Peter heard everything what bobby said about him he felt guilty)

Bobby: "there you are peter"

Peter: "hey babe you ok did you enjoy your hen do"

Bobby: "yeah did you my husband to be"

Perter: "yeah it was good thanks, you won't believe who turned up"

Bobby: "can I have a guess"

Peter: "yeah, but you won't get it"

Bobby: "was it your school mate Dan M"

Peter: "well yeah how did you know that?"

Bobby: "because I told him to come and surprise you"

Peter: "oh ok that was nice of you"

Bobby: "are you sure you ok, you can tell me anything you know"

Peter: "no am fine honesty, just stop asking if am alright"

(Peter runs upstairs and closes the bedroom door behind him)

Scene 12

(Peter is on the phone to Dan M)

Peter: "why did you lie and said you were just passing by well you know bobby invited you"

Dan M: "because what you did to me you kissed my girlfriend in school and couple weeks ago before your stag do"

Peter: "it was a mistake I'm happy now with bobby leave me alone I don't want you in my life no more.

Dan M: "fine ok then bye then, but I hope he finds out before the wedding"

Peter: "who?"

Dan M: "your husband to be bobby"

(Bobby heard everything from outside the bedroom door)

Peter: "he will never find out"

(Bobby opens the bedroom door and he says)

Bobby: "I know how can you do this to me we are about to get married and you kissed Dan M girlfriend couple days before you stag do"

Peter: "please it was a mistake I love you it was just the one time, she means nothing to me you do"

(Bobby walks over to peter and slaps him over the face)

Bobby: "don't ever call me your mysterious boy ever again I never want to see your face again"

(Bobby packs his bag and moves in with his mam again)

Peter: "please don't leave me I love you"

Bobby: "I told you downstairs if you want to tell me anything you can, you could of told me then not when Dan was on the phone how can I trust you again"

(Bobby opens the front door and slams it behind him leaving the key behind)

Charlotte and Leanne: "how can you do this to bobby peter he loves you with all his heart and you do something like that"

(The girls slaps peter over his face leaving with bobby)

Peter: "aaaaaahhhhhh how can I have done this to bobby I love him, I've just lost the love of my life"

(Peter smashes glasses on the floor)

Scene 13

(There was a knock on bobby's mam's house)

Lynne: "what is wrong bobby what happened?"

Bobby: he cheated on me with a girl how can he do this to me"

(Bobby fell on the floor with a broken heart)

Lynne: "Anna and Matthew can I have some help please"

Anna and Matthew: "what's up?"

Lynne: "come quick please"

(Lynne, Anna and Matthew picked bobby up of the floor)

Anna: "what's happened bobby"

Bobby: "well he was on the phone to Dan M and he said to peter about how peter kissed his girlfriend at school and couple days before his stag do"

Lynne and Anna: "what how can he do that to you"

Matthew: "I know that Dan M was trouble"

Bobby: "what did say Matthew?"

Matthew: "nothing"

Bobby: "no you said that Dan M was trouble what you mean by that"

Matthew: "well…… on the stag do we were playing a game and Dan M said how peter kissed his girlfriend a couple days before the stag do"

Bobby: "how long have you known this for please don't tell me you have known a long time"

Matthew: well I just told ya since the stag do"

Bobby: "get out of my face I never want to see you again"

(Bobby runs off to his secret place which is the tree house with rose gold glitter in)

Scene 14

(Bobby is writing his new song about how he is feeling)

(Lynne, Anna and Matthew where looking for bobby)

(Lynne was on the top floor looking and shouting)

Lynne: "come on son we can talk about this are you up here am your mother talk to me"

(Anna was on the 2nd floor)

Anna: "come on bobby talk to auntie Anna if you don't want to talk to your mam"

(Matthew was on the first floor)

Matthew: "come on bro where are you we can sort this out together"

(Couple minutes later Matthew had an idea where he was and he looked in the tree house)

Matthew: "bobby there you are we all looking for you come on we supposed to be like brothers"

(Anna and Lynne saw from in the window)

Bobby: "well if we are like supposed to be brother I can't believe my supposed brother just stabs me in the back because I'm heartbroken about you knowing about the kiss and you not telling me"

Matthew: "well I did but I wanted you to find out yourself would you believe me if I did tell you"

Bobby: "true am sorry what I said I was just upset and shouldn't take it on you"

Matthew: "it's ok I'm always going to be here for you that was brothers are for"

Bobby: "true"

(They hugged it out)

(Anna and Lynne where crying with emotions)

Anna: "lynne pass me the tissue"

(Lynne passed the tissues to Anna)

Lynne: "Anna pass me the popcorn please it's just a brotherly love

(Bobby and Matthew were laughing there heads of in the tree)

Scene 15

(Couple weeks later there is a knock on bobby's house door)

(Knock knock knock knock)

(Bobby looks at the window, and it is peter who he sees)

Bobby: "what the hell is he doing here, mam peter is here"

Peter: "I'm a fool for bobby I love you I made a mistake please come back to me"

(Lynne and Anna opens the door)

Anna: "you cheating bastard how could you"

Peter: "I deserve everything I get ok"

Lynne: "you"

(Lynne punches peter in the face, peter falls on the floor)

(Peter sees bobby)

Peter: "bobby please speak to me hear what I have to say please"

Bobby: "fine ok"

(Peter comes in the house)

(Matthew and peter starts to fight)

Matthew: "how could you hurt bobby like that"

Peter: "it was a mistake I told you that"

Bobby: "Matthew will you leave the room please we are having a private word"

Matthew: "fine I will"

(Peter starts to speak will tears from his eyes)

Peter: "bobby I'm sorry I was stupid and it was wrong I love you and no one else"

Bobby: "how can I start trusting you again I loved you, you were my world?"

Peter: "I wish you didn't invite Dan M because none of this would of happened"

Bobby: "I would have known somehow what you did"

Peter: "your right so what do you want to do, do you want to call of the wedding"

Bobby: "no I don't want to do that"

Peter: "what"

Bobby: "no I want to still marry you because I love you but I need to know you not going to cheat on me again"

Peter: - "I won't I promise I love you so much and the person you have become you are so amazing and for giving me another chance"

Bobby: "fine last chance now, I'll be staying home for another week on my own though ok"

Peter: "ok I love you"

(Peter left to go back home to America)

Bobby: "peter will you ask Matthew to come in the room please "

Peter: "ok, Matthew bobby wants you"

Matthew: "ok peter"

Scene 16

(Matthew walks in the room)

Matthew: "yes bobs what you want"

Bobby: "I want you and me to murder Dan M

Matthew: am in after what he has done to you and peter and also am so glad you both worked it out"

Bobby: "thanks it means a lot now murder plan how do you want us to kill Dan M then Matthew I think we should throw McDonalds burger at him till he drowns in them like a pool of water what do you think"

(Matthew had a plan on how killing Dan M)

Matthew: "how about you ring Dan M up to say you want me and you to go and speak to him about

something then we both go in his fridge and take his crunchies bars and eat them in-front of him so he faints then we will kill him with a pillow fight, then dig him in a hole when he has died"

Bobby: "you know what Matthew let's do it"

Scene 17

(Bobby rings up Dan M to see if he can come round to speak to him)

Dan M: "hello who is this?"

Bobby: "hi Dan is bobby I was wondering if I can come over your flat to speak to you please

Dan M: "yeah no problem how about 12 tomorrow dinner time"

Bobby: "great see you then"

(Bobby and Matthew turns up to Dan's M flat)

(Knock knock)

Dan M: "hello bobby, huh hello Matthew"

(Matthew ties Dan M up on the chair and gag him with tea towel)

Bobby: "Matthew"

Matthew: "yeah bobby"

Bobby: "I fancy going into Dan M fridge to see what he has got"

Matthew: "yeah me too lets go and see what we can eat"

(Bobby opens the fridge door)

Bobby: "Matthew you see what I see"

Matthew: "oh yeah"

Bobby and Matthew: "oh yeah crunchies"

(Matthew and bobby eat the last two bars of the crunchies bar)

Matthew and bobby: "yum yum in my tummy"

(Dan M is trying to scream for help)

Bobby: "what Dan M we can't hear you"

(Matthew and bobby get a pillow each and start hitting it to him)

(10 minutes later we felt Dan M pulse to see if he was alive and he wasn't)

Matthew: "bobby lets go bury a hole in his garden"

Bobby: "ok am up for that"

(We buried him in his garden so no one will ever find out where he is)

Since 17

(Matthew said to bobby)

Matthew: "we have to hide the evidence bobby you put the crunchies wrapper in the sink and I will sort out the body.

(Bobby and Matthew put the body in Matthew bubble gum colour fiat 500, Dan M is dead and tied while we are driving to the location bobby and Matthew are singing to bring me to heaven by Svanescence.

(Bobby came up with the plan where to hide the body)

Bobby: "Matthew"?

Matthew: "yes mate what's up"?

Bobby: "why don't we hide the body in toys r us it's a mint location he will be with the all the toys that he likes just as star wars, star trek and marvel".

Matthew: "you know what bobby why do you always come up with all the good ideas".

Bobby: "because I have the brains lol"

(Bobby and Mathew went to the location, Matthew opened the boot)

Matthew: "hurry up booby stop putting your make up on and help me with this body"

Bobby: chill out hold your hair on am coming".

Matthew: "well instead of putting your make up on come and help me take this body in"

Bobby: "ok"

(Bobby and Matthew got the body out of the car)

Matthew and bobby: "one two three lift"

(Matthew and bobby opened the doors to toys r us)

Matthew and bobby: "wow this place is scary dark"

(Matthew and bobby are scared of the dark)

Bobby: "Matthew"

Matthew: "what"

Bobby: "I'm scared of the dark"

Matthew: "me too, but we have to finish the work off"

Bobby: "ok"

(Matthew and bobby where digging up the floor to but Dan M in)

Matthew: "hurry up bobby this place gives me the scare"

Bobby: "I'm going as fast as we can"

(Matthew and bobby completed the task)

Bobby: "hurry up Matthew we got to go now we done what we wanted to do"

Matthew: "ok bobby coming now"

(Bobby and Matthew were running to the exit and they heard a noise and you won't believe what it was)

Matthew: "bobby did you hear that"

Bobby: "yeah I hope I am wrong"

Berbie: "hello boys I saw what you did and am going to tell on you"

Matthew and bobby: "aaaaaahhhhh! Let's see you try you toy"

Berbie: "am going to kill you both for killing that man"

Matthew and bobby: "hahahahaha try it!

(Berbie was attacking bobby and Matthew)

Bobby: "Ouch"

Matthew: "take that you toy"

(Matthew attacked the Berbie with a bat and before Matthew took the batteries out the Berbie was talking to bobby)

Berbie: "please bobby don't let him take my battery out I'm sorry"

Bobby: "Matthew look at him we can't take his battery out"

Matthew: "WHAT ARE YOU JOKING ME HE TRIED TO KILL US"

Bobby: "I know but just look at him"

(Bobby took the Berbie off Matthew and then the Berbie was biting bobby's arms)

Bobby: "OUCH MATTHEW TAKE THEM OUT NOW PLEASE"

(Matthew took the batteries out)

<u>Scene 18</u>

(Bobby and Matthew were driving back home listening to murder on the dancefloor)

(2 weeks later it was the wedding for bobby and peter)

(Bobby stayed at the hotel they were getting married out they got married at Judge in Barm bobby took the girls and the boys stayed at peter's and bobby's house)

(Bobby kissed peter and said)

Bobby: "I see you tomorrow for our big day Hun"

Peter: "I love you see you tomorrow for our big day can't wait to see you in the morning"

Bobby: "can't wait"

(Peter got bobby a massive party bus the colour was rose gold glitter just what bobby like with drinks and cocktails and gins and a pole and smoking machine and bubbles)

(Bobby and the girls went outside and bobby says)

Bobby: "what the hell is this?"

Peter: "surprise I love you"

Bobby: "I love you too thanks babes (crying)

Peter: "you're welcome"

(Bobby and all the girls went to the hotel to stay over)

(Charlotte and Leanne were playing on the tunes since Leanne worked on the bar and Charlotte was working as a DJ)

(They played songs like Bobby Latheron, Britney opears, Vengbears, Char, Bqua and of cause, they played Peter Sande)

(Bobby was talking to his maid of honor Suzy about what time the hairdresser was coming)

Bobby: "Suzy what time is Nicky Blarke"

Suzy: "he is all booked in for 8"

Bobby: "great thanks girl"

(Bobby and the make-up artist Natalie were practice for how long it will take to get ready for the big day tomorrow)

Bobby: "Natalie will you do a practice for tomorrow please so we don't rush with time babe"

Natalie: "of cause we can"

(Natalie asked bobby what colour lipstick and lip liner on)

Natalie: "so bobby what colour lipstick and lip liner do you want on"

Bobby: "can I have my usually colour please nude please darl"

(Natalie shouted at bobby and said)

Natalie: "you always go for the nude why do you always go for the NUDE COLOUR"

Bobby: "because darling I want to look natural and good looking ok"

Natalie: "ok babe I'll do it for you"

(Natalie did step by step what she was putting on bobby)

Natalie: "so bobby what is your skin like wet or do you get dry skin so I know what kind of foundation to put on you"

Bobby: "I get really dry skin"

Natalie: "I have got the perfect foundation for you it's by fabulous make-up"

Bobby: "ohhhh gimme gimme but it on me girl"

Natalie: "ok, now we have finished the foundation we going to but some pounder on your face just to make you glow, then we going to but on the nude lipstick but it stays on all day and the nude lip liner, then we going to but some on nude glitter eyeshadow and a clear mascara because your eyelashes are so long and shamzing and so gorgeous".

Bobby: "thanks babe"

(It took over an hour to put the make up on)

Natalie: "ok bobby you can turn around now"

(Bobby turned around on his rose gold glitter chair and said)

Bobby: "OMG girl you made me look shinini for my wedding day thank you babe"

Natalie: "you welcome babe am glad you like it"

(The girls and bobby were drinking gins all night and having pillow fights and games)

(Peter asked Matthew something)

Peter: "Matthew"

Matthew: "yes Peter what do you want"

Peter: "Matthew will you be my best man please at my wedding"

Matthew: "of cause I will be peter and thank you"

(Matthew ranged Suzy up)

Matthew: Suzy you won't believe what peter asked me to be"

Suzy: "what babes"

Matthew: "he asked me to be his best man for the wedding"

Suzy: "aaahh bobby peter asked Matthew to be his best man"

Bobby: "aaahh am so pleased he asked him"

(Bobby asked his mam something and Anna at the same time)

Bobby: "mam and Anna will you do me a big favour tomorrow please"

Lynne and Anna: "what the matter bobby"

Bobby: "well mam and Anna I want you both to be both on my side while am going to the aisle is that ok with you both am asking you Anna because I don't have a dad and you are like a father figure to me"

(Anna and Lynne started to cry like they usually do)

Bobby: "stop please don't cry everytime I try to do something nice for you both!"

Lynne and Anna: "ok"

(Leanne had a surprise for bobby)

Leanne: "bobby guess who is coming tomorrow!"

Bobby: "who"

Leanne: "my husband Bradley Looper"

Bobby: "aaaahhh can't wait to see him like"

(Then charlotte had a surprise for bobby)

Charlotte: "ohhhh bobby guess who is coming to sing at your wedding!"

Bobby: "who please tell me it's your husband chad"

Charlotte: "well yeah it is how you knew"

Bobby: "aaahh please tell me he is going to do my favourite song for my 1st dance with peter called never gonna be alone"

Charlotte: "he will do any song you ask him"

Bobby: "aaahh thanks babe's xx"

Charlotte: "you welcome darl"

Scene 19

(The big day for bobby and peter)

(Bobby and all the girls were getting ready and listening to music with a bottle of bubble)

Suzy: "Natalie where is the hairdresser he is five minutes late"

Natalie: "it's ok Suzy I ring him now"

Suzy: "thanks"

(Natalie rang up the hairdresser)

Natalie: "hello Nicky where the hell are you"

Nicky: "am so sorry traffic is bad am five minutes away"

(Bobby was on the toilet and didn't see the time or he would have been panicking)

(Nicky arrived 5 minutes like he said)

(Natalie and Suzy went to go and meet him in the reception)

Natalie and Suzy: "hi Nicky you need to run run run upstairs bobby is on the toilet so go go"

(Nicky just made it on time and then bobby came out of the toilet)

Nicky: "so am guessing you're the lucky man"

Bobby: "yeah I am thanks"

Nicky: "so bobby what do you want me to do your hair"

Bobby: "I want my hair purple grey if you know what I mean"

Nicky: "I do"

(2 hours later and 2-hour till the wedding)

Nicky: "bobby you can turn around now"

Bobby: "oh wow thank you so much I love it so much thank you"

Nicky: "you very welcome"

Bobby: "won't you like to stay for the wedding"

Nicky: "are you sure that would be great thanks"

Bobby: "you very welcome"

(Bobby got the photography to take some pictures of all the girls)

Bobby: "dani will you take some pictures of me and the girls please chick"

Dani: "yeah am coming now"

(Dani told the girls and bobby how to stand)

Dani: 1st "now girls look at bobby's gorgeous ring and look shock bobby look glamour"

2nd "now bobby looks outside the window or sit on the balcony of the window looking to the sky"

3rd "now everyone look like a diva like you all are"

Scene 20

(Peter and all the guess are all waiting for bobby to come through the doors)

(The song bobby as choosing for the brides to go down was single badies)

(These are the orders who went down the aisle first)

1st Suzy and Natalie

2nd Leanne and charlotte

(Then the registrar said now ladies and gentlemen can we all stand up for the groom)

(Then came with rusty baby pink suit on and he came down the aisle with his arm Lynne with left arm and Anna with the right arm with the song by bobby Latheron – happy ending)

The registrar: "ladies and gentleman you now can take your seat"

(Everyone sat down)

(The registrar starts to speak)

(When bobby turned he was shocked who was marrying myself and peter it was Char)

(Bobby screamed)

"Aaaahhh its Char OMG I love you so much I would love it if you can only sing one of my songs in the wedding"

Char: "of cause now may I finish what I came to do"

Bobby: "yeah sorry people"

(Char starts to speak)

"Peter you can now say your vows"

"I take you to be my husband. To have to hold from this day forward for better, for worse, for richer, for poorer, in sickness and in health, to love to cherish, till death do us part, according to god's holy law; and this is my solemn vow".

(Peter had to say that)

Char: "Now bobby it's your turn to do your speech"

Bobby: "I promise to never watch the next episode on Netflix without you, no matter how much I want to"

(Everyone started to laugh)

(Then we got married)

<u>Scene 21</u>

(Everyone was waiting to throw rose gold glitter confetti at the grooms)

(Everyone cheered when they came out)

(They all got on the field to take a picture of everyone)

(Then everyone just went on they own way)

(The photography dani said to bobby and peter)

"Can I take your wedding pictures now just the two of us and we said yeah"

(So bobby, dani and peter went for an hour to take some pictures)

(Bobby and peter had the e-cig with them bobby had a rose gold glitter one and peter had a black one)

(So dani said)

"Can you both look at each other and do a love heart with your clouds with you e cig"

Bobby and peter: "we can try yeah"

(The pictures looked amazing)

Bobby: "I love them thanks"

Peter: "thank you dani"

(We finished the pictures and it was time to get pictures with our family)

(Peter was the only child and his parents died before meeting me, so we got pictures of my family with him in and all the pictures were amazing)

(Then all the girls and bobby got they pictures done)

Bobby: "hurry up girls where are you lol"

Girls: "we are coming xx"

(The pictures dani took of me and the girls were amazing and there was some funny pics)

(And then it was the lads turn and they pictures were funny)

<u>Scene 22</u>

(After the pictures where done we all sat on the tables they were rose gold glitter all over such as flowers knife and forks etc.)

(Then me and peter were giving our presents out who helped at the wedding)

(Bobby spoken)

Bobby: "ladies and gentlemen we didn't get everyone a present but you are all welcome to our brand new villa in Las Vegas for a week"

Boys and girls: "aaaaaahhhhh yeahhh baby"

(Then it was time for the speeches, bobby went first)

Bobby: "the first time I met peter, I couldn't take my eyes of him, and then when he was singing my songs my heart skipped a beat lol, he was shy to ask me out so I asked him out, but I know we had our ups and downs but I can't imagine my life without him".

(Then it was peters turn to tell his speech)

Peter: "when I first met bobby when I opened the door I was like wow he is nice looking, then when we started to work with each other I started to have feeling but couldn't tell him, so when bobby asked me out I was like walking in the sky, because I've been waiting for someone like you to walk into my life, I know we had our ups and downs but we are more stronger than ever".

(Bobby started to cry) "I love you"

Peter: "I love you too"

Scene 23

(Couple hours later)

(Charlotte said to bobby)

Charlotte:" bobby come here want you to meet someone"

Bobby: "please tell me it's your husband chad"

Charlotte: "yeah it is"

Bobby: "where is he then?"

Charlotte: "over here quick"

(Bobby and chad met for the first time)

Bobby: "wow your good looking you charlotte you got a keeper here like babe"

Charlotte: "I know I have babe"

(Chad says to bobby)

Chad: "I really like your music bobby very strong words I hear would you find if I bring one of your songs out"

(Bobby started to cry)

Bobby: "really you want to sing one of my songs, yes yes yes let's do it"

(Bobby asked chad to sing one of his songs for the wedding for the first dance)

Chad: "yes I would love to which one would you like me to sing"

Bobby: "nobody knows"

Chad: "yes that's my favorite song ever"

Bobby: "omg"

<u>Scene 24</u>

(Leanne asked bobby something)

Leanne: "bobby come here and meet my husband"

Bobby: "where is he brad brad brad?"

Leanne: "he is over here quick"

(Bobby and brad met the first time)

Bobby: "wow you are a diamond look at you"

Leanne: "I know I am one lucky girl aren't I babe"

Bobby: "yeah babe"

(Bradley asked bobby if he liked to go and see someone)

Bradley: "it's a surprise come with me"

Bobby: "ohhhh ok am coming"

(Bradley took bobby to see that person and you won't believe who it was)

(Bradley was talking to the woman)

Bobby: "aaaaaahhhhh it's lady baba"

Lady baba: "congrats on your wedding bobby"

Bobby: "thanks lady baba omg you both here it's like a dream"

(Lady Baba and Bradley asked bobby a question)

Lady baba and Bradley: "can we do a movie about your life"

Bobby: "what really really"

Lady baba and Bradley: "yeah really really"

Bobby: "yeah omg yeah"

Scene 25

(Me and peter were ready for the first dance, and chad was singing it was amazing. Then bobby and peter say to each other)

Bobby and peter: "this has been the best day of our life's"

(Then we cut our cake out it was of cause rose gold glitter cake everyone cheered when we cut into the cake)

(Then charlotte played some good tunes as the dj)

(Then peter called rick to come and play with his guitar and he played livin on a nightmare)

(Then it was time to go to bed in our honeymoon room)

Scene 26

(3 months later bobby and peter went on the honeymoon to the Greece)

(Bobby had to ask peter something)

Bobby: "Hunny buns have you ever thought about having kids"

Peter: "yeah of cause I have but was waiting for you to ask me if you wanted any"

Bobby: "yeah of cause I want children"

(Peter and bobby kissed to celebrate they news)

(Bobby and peter went to see bobby's family to tell them the news)

(Bobby starts to speak)

Bobby: "hi guys got some good news we like to tell you all"

Bobby's family: "WHAT"

Bobby and peter: "we want to make a family"

Bobby's family: "AAAAHHHH"

(Everyone congrats the couples)

4 weeks later

(Bobby and peter went for meeting to see if anyone would like to be our surrogate, but no one really they liked)

Bobby: "peter what we are going to do no one we really like"

Peter: "it's ok honey am sure someone will come to us we going to like"

5 weeks later

(Bobby got a call from one of his friends)

Bobby: "hello who is speaking please?"

Dani dye: "it's me dani?"

Bobby: "hi dani how are you?"

Dani: "I was thinking it is up to you and peter, I would be honoured to be your surrogate"

Bobby: "are you sure about this, I just ask peter now, honey can you come here please"

Peter: "coming darling"

Bobby: "I've got dani on the phone and she want to be our surrogate, what do you think?"

Peter: "yeah let's do it with dani we know her and she is our friend"

Bobby and peter: "yeah defo dani and thank you"

(Bobby told the family they have got a surrogate and they were all pleased)

(Bobby and peter wanted to know what they were having and they were having a little girl)

(Bobby and peter were so happy)

(8 months in the pregnancy)

(Bobby and peter had a baby shower what our friends and family did for them)

(Then the baby came 4 weeks early but sadly it died in stillborn)

Bobby and peter and family and friends went to the funeral)

Bobby: "noooo why can't it be me"

Peter: "it's ok honey, it's hard but we are strong"

Bobby: "I know darling love you"

Peter: "love you too"

<u>Scene 27</u>

(Peter couldn't cope with the loss of our baby girl so he turned to drinking for comfort)

(Bobby hide all the drinks in the house)

Bobby: "what the hell is this peter?"

Peter: "what do you think it is stupid?"

Bobby: "who the hell do you think you're calling stupid I lost my child as well not just you"

Peter: "whatever"

Bobby: "you know what I know it's hard for the both of us we need to get some help ok"

Peter: "I agree with you"

<u>Scene 28</u>

(On the day we got the counseling)

Counselor: "Hello my name is Angela, how can I help you both"

Bobby: "hello there my name is bobby and this is my husband peter we lost our child at still birth we both are upset about I still, but my husband is drinking to forget about it".

Counselor: "well am sorry for your lost, I can't make you forget I can make you heal"

Peter: "great thank you am ready for the challenge"

Counselor: "great let's get started"

(6 weeks later)

Counselor: "great I think you both done really well in these 6 weeks it's now to end the counseling but remember you 2 love for each other that's all you did is love"

Peter and bobby: "thank you I feel I can heal now"

(Bobby and peter got the Counselor some rose gold glitter flowers to say thank you)

Counselor: "thank you both you didn't have too"

Peter: "no we wanted to"

Scene 29

(2 years later)

(Bobby's been thinking about doing a book)

Bobby: "what shall I do my book about, I might do my book about life with autism, script and my music lyrics"

Peter: "what you doing my darling"

Bobby: "thinking of selling a book I might go to an author"

(Bobby looks up an author online to sell his book with him)

Bobby: "he looks alright and he has good review and 5 star"

(Bobby rings up the author)

Bobby: "hello my name is bobby what is your name"

Author: "hello my name is Hugh Hackman nice to meet you bobby what can I do for you"

Bobby: "well I have done this book and wondered if I can come over to yours and show you it if that is ok"

Hugh: "yeah no problem do you fancy meeting up for a coffee first about your interest and why you want to write this book"

Bobby: "yeah, do you know where the peppermill café is"

Hugh: "yeah I do"

Bobby: "good do you fancy meeting up on the 23rd of June 2019"

Hugh: "yeah great is 12 ok with you"

Bobby: "yeah see you then"

Scene 30

(The day has arrived to meet up to chat about my book)

(Bobby ordered his food parmo, chips and salad)

(Hugh walked in and ordered his food)

Hugh: "hello are you bobby"

Bobby: "well yes you must be Hugh Hackman"

Hugh: "yes so well what can I do for you?"

Bobby: "well my name is bobby, I write my own songs which I have a contact and I love working with celebrities, my songs are very open and I just want to get my words out and how I feel, I have started thinking about writing a book about autism because I want people to understand about people how they live and how they cope day to day, so am here if you can help me if you would just go through it to see if it makes sense or spells checks"

Hugh: "well I would love too also I have listened to your songs and I love them that much and I wondered if it be ok with you, we are doing the greatest programme 2 and wondered if we can sing some of your songs"

Bobby: "yes please if you don't mind, because I want my songs all over the place and it would help me so much, and thank you"

Hugh: "you welcome, would you like to come on set and meet people and see what we do"

Bobby: "yeah if you don't mind"

Hugh: "and of course I will help you with your book and I will bring it out for you"

Bobby: "thank you so much it will help so much people" (crying)

Hugh: "shall we go then on this big adventure"

Bobby: "yeah I'll just ring my husband and tell him the good news"

Hugh: "ok"

Scene 31

(We went onto the set of the greatest programme 2)

Bobby: "wow this is like a dream come true, I can't wait for my song to be on here"

Hugh: "bobby you want to meet the cast of the show"

Bobby: "yes please if you don't mind"

Hugh: "of course it's no problem"

(Bobby met the cast and they all welcomed him and said)

The cast: "bobby how are you, we all welcome you here, I think you are a amazing what you do, and I really love your songs"

Bobby: "well thank you, I can't wait to see who is gonna sing my songs"

Hugh: "bobby am gonna take you to meet my family if that's ok"

Bobby: "yeah ok"

(Bobby's been working with Hugh now for 9 months)

Scene 32

(The day bobby meet the family)

Hugh's mam: "hello there you must be bobby, Hugh told us everything about you"

Hugh's sister jess: "omg I love your songs they are amazing you are my biggest fan"

Hugh sister Jessie: "I really love what you are doing, you are amazing keep it up"

Bobby: "thank you all, and I hope whatever he has told you it's all good LOL"

Kate: "and I am Hugh's wife"

Bobby: "hello nice to meet you"

(Later on bobby heard the mam and the new sister talking)

The mam: "are we gonna tell bobby how he feels"

Jess: "I don't know"

Jessie: "am going to tell bobby, I hate his wife me"

The mam: "we all hate her LOL"

(Bobby over hear what they are saying)

Bobby: "is everything ok"

Jessie: "well we got to tell you something"

Bobby: "what"

Jess: "well mam do you want to tell him"

Bobby: "will someone tell me what's going on"

The mam: well, my son really likes you"

Bobby: "well I like him too"

The mam: "no he really really likes you, if you know what I mean"

Bobby: "I have to go sorry, peter I got to go bye"

(Bobby slams the door)

Scene 33

(The next day Hugh rang up bobby and said)

Hugh: "why did you leave last night dead quick"

Bobby: "I need to speak to you meet me in my car in half an hour"

Hugh: "ok?"

(Half an hour came up)

Bobby: "Hugh I'm over here get in"

Hugh: "ok coming in now?

(Hugh got in the car)

Hugh: "what is wrong with you bobby you acting all strange"

Bobby: "I know you know"

Hugh: "you know what"

Bobby: "you fancy me"

(Hugh looked shocked)

Hugh: "how do you know that?"

Bobby: "your family told me"

Hugh: "it's true I'm sorry I know you're married but it's true I like….

(Bobby kissed Hugh)

Hugh: "does this mean you like me too"

Bobby: "yeah I'm so sorry, I've like you since I've seen you"

Hugh: "why didn't you tell me?"

Bobby: "telling a straight man you like him sounds a bit silly lol"

Hugh: "true lol"

(They kissed again)

(But what they didn't know is that Hugh wife is watching them)

(Hugh wife rings up bobby's husband)

Hugh wife: "hello is this peter"

Peter: "yeah hello who am I talking to please?"

Hugh wife: "I am Hugh wife"

Peter: "oh hello nice to meet you what can I help you with please?"

Hugh wife: "well did you know your husband is having an affair with my husband"

Peter: "what how do you know this"

Hugh wife: "because I've just seen them and I've got a picture of them now, I will send you it now"

Peter: "ok"

(Beep beep)

Peter: "how can bobby do this to me?"

(Peter and Hugh wife come up with a plan to kill them)

Scene 34

(Bobby walked in while peter was on the phone with Hugh's wife)

Bobby: "OMG HE KNOWS"

(Bobby close the door behind him so quite that peter didn't hear)

(Bobby rings up Hugh)

Bobby: "THEY KNOW THEY KNOW"

Peter: "they know what"

Bobby: "what we did, they want to kill us"

Hugh: "ok bobby where are you"

Bobby: "am driving to my mam's can you meet me there"

Hugh: "yeah"

(Hugh and bobby went to bobby's mams house)

Bobby: "MAM MAM MAM"

Lynne Anna Matthew Suzy: "AHHHHHH WE LOVE YOU"

Bobby: "yeah yeah we all know he is we both in danger can you help us"

Lynee: "what's happened like?"

Bobby: "wellllll, we kissed"

Matthew and Suzy: "yeah about time"

Lynee and Anna: "get in there"

Bobby: "you're not mad then"

Everyone: "no"

Bobby: "his wife and my husband kind of know and they want to kill us what shall we do"

Matthew: "why don't we all just pack all our bags and move somewhere where they can't find us"

Scene 35

(They all packs they bags bobby went home and Hugh went home)

(While Hugh packed his bag his wife given him a drink)

Hugh wife: "darling I made you a drink"

Hugh: "thank you darling I'll have it now"

(She put poison in his drink)

Hugh: "whhhaaatttttt whoa what have you done to me"

(He was on the phone to bobby at the time)

Bobby: "darling you ok"

Hugh wife: "I killed him and you will be next"

Bobby: "aaaahhh why have you killed him"

Hugh wife's: "because he choose you, he was gonna run away with you"

Bobby: "you bitch I hate you so much"

(Bobby is packing his bags quick)

Peter: "where you think you going"

Bobby: "you drinking man, I tried to help you but I did to think about myself, so I'm going back home sorry"

Peter: "oh no you're not"

(Peter attacks bobby, but bobby escaped and ran to the car and drives off)

Scene 36

(Bobby was driving as he can, listening to his new song "wake me up")

Bobby: "tell me I'm in a bad dream please aaaaaahhhhhh"

(Peter catches up to bobby)

Peter: "you're not going anywhere"

Bobby: "you need to leave me alone right now"

Peter: "you are an ass I'm going to kill you"

Bobby: "Peter please don't, just go away please"

(Bobby lose control of the car, the car went upside down)

(Bobby rings his family)

(Ring ring ring ring)

(Bobby mam answers the phone but it on speaker)

Lynne: "bobby where are you"

Bobby: "mam, guys I'm sorry love you all"

Matthew: "what's going on?"

(Peter comes on the phone and says)

Peter: "I've killed him"

Matthew: "nooooo"

Lynne: "you leave him alone you monster"

Bobby: "bye guys"

(Peter walks off)

(Lynne and the gang go looking for bobby's car they found it)

(Everyone sees bobby dead)

Everyone: "nooooo" (crying)

Lynne: "we all got to be strong now, we need to sort out the funeral"

Anna: "ok, if I known bobby he would want rose gold glitter coffin"

Suzy: "you're right lol"

Scene 37

(The day of the funeral)

(People did they speech and they goodbyes)

Lynee: (crying)

Matthew: "come on Lynne bobby wouldn't want to see you like this"

Lynee: "ok you're right"

(Everyone left)

Matthew: "bye mate see ya one day"

(1 hour later when everyone left)

(scratch scratch scratch)

(Bobby came out of the coffin)

Bobby: "heeeeeellllppppp me please someone"

Matthew: "who was that, it sound like it keep back from back there I'll go and check"

Bobby: "Matthew help me please"

Matthew: "bobby"

(Matthew falls on the ground)

(Bobby wakes Matthew up)

Bobby: "mate you ok"

Matthew: "omg you're alive"

Bobby: "mate I had to fake my death because he would of killed me if I didn't"

(Matthew shouted for help)

Matthew: "hhhhheeeeeellllpppppp us please"

(Lynne Anna Suzy runs of to Matthew)

Bobby: "hi guys"

(They all fall on the floor)

Bobby: "really guys get up, I had to fake it so he couldn't kill me"

Lynne: "but we saw you dead"

Bobby: "I'm a good actor mother please"

Anna: "his got a point there"

(Bobby laugh but in pain)

Scene 38

Suzy: "we got to ring the ambulance"

Matthew: "I'll do it"

(Ambulance came and they but bobby in a hospital bed to get scan so he hasn't broke anything)

Bobby: "Matthew ring the police please"

Matthew: "ok I'm on it"

PC Amy: "hi there bobby I'm PC Amy now what happened here"

Bobby: "my husband tried to kill me, because I was having an affair with someone else"

PC Amy: "wow that I new story, I thought you had died"

Bobby: "I had to fake my own death because he was going to kill me"

PC Amy: "ok you didn't do the right thing but you safe have you broken any bones"

Bobby: "I'm just waiting for the results"

(The nurse comes in)

Nurse poppy sunflower: "hi bobby I've got your results in you just bruised yourself you're lucky to be alive you be fine by tomorrow"

Bobby: "thank you nurse"

(Bobby was telling PC Vicky something)

Bobby: "please can I go and see Hugh, his wife killed him"

Matthew Suzy Anna Lynne: "no way you ok bobby"

Bobby: "I just want to see goodbye to him on my own"

(So Matthew took bobby to see Hugh grave)

Scene 39

Bobby: "Matthew you can leave me here will you wait here for me"

Matthew: "yeah no problem"

Bobby: "cheers"

(Bobby goes to the grave)

Bobby: "I can't believe I'm saying goodbye to you like this, I hope we will be together soon when it's my turn, I love you, I know it's too late to tell you but I do"

(Bobby walks off crying and he hears a thing)

(knock knock knock)

Bobby: "WHAT THE HELL"

Hugh: "I love you too"

Bobby: "is that you Hugh"

Hugh: "yeah"

(Bobby scratches the floor with his wedding ring)

Bobby: "I'm coming now wait there"

(Bobby got him out of the grave)

Hugh: "I love you"

Bobby: "what we gonna do now"

Hugh: "well I know what to do get your family I get mine and we all live in Las Vegas you fancy it baby"

Bobby: "hell yeah, but what we going to do about them two"

(Ring ring ring ring)

(Matthew is ringing bobby up)

Bobby: "mate he is alive"

Matthew: "well never he is an actor you know"

Bobby: "true, now what do you want to tell me"

Matthew: "They have arrested the wife and peter"

(Bobby and peter kissed)

Scene 40

(The day of court of Hugh wife and peter)

(Bobby Lynne Matthew Suzy Anna and Hugh turned up to see what they were gonna get)

(Judge Chris franks thought and he knew what he was gonna say)

Judge Chris franks: "peter and hugh ex-wife shall we say now you both going down for the rest of your life for trying to kill you're husbands"

(Everyone cheered)

Everyone: "yesss"

Peter: "I thought you died I saw you die"

Bobby: "that's what you call a good actor try again you ass, watch this Hugh"

(Bobby kisses Hugh)

Hugh ex-wife: "you ass I will killed you"

Hugh: "duh am alive you bitch hahahaha watch this"

(Hugh kisses bobby)

(Bobby Hugh and family lived happily ever after and they had a child called Shannon a girl in last Vegas hospital)

(The end)

Lightning Source UK Ltd.
Milton Keynes UK
UKHW051029101219
355101UK00008B/129/P